D0907202

Koss's Cytology of the Urinary Tract
with Histopathologic Correlations

Leopold G. Koss · Rana S. Hoda

Koss's Cytology of the Urinary Tract with Histopathologic Correlations

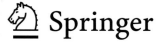 Springer

Leopold G. Koss, MD, Doct. HC (multiple)
Distinguished Professor University Emeritus
Montefiore Medical Center
Albert Einstein College of Medicine
Bronx, NY USA

Rana S. Hoda, MD, FIAC
Professor of Pathology and Director of
Papanicolaou Cytology Laboratory
Department of Pathology and Laboratory Medicine
New York Presbyterian Hospital
Weill Cornell Medical College
New York, NY USA

ISBN 978-1-4614-2055-2   e-ISBN 978-1-4614-2056-9
DOI 10.1007/978-1-4614-2056-9
Springer New York Dordrecht Heidelberg London

Library of Congress Control Number: 2011944181

Printed on acid-free paper

Springer is part of Springer Science+Business Media (www.springer.com)

Foreword

"One picture is Worth a Thousand Words (一畫勝千言)" is an ancient Chinese proverb; that captures the essence of this book "Koss's Cytology of the Urinary Tract with Histopathologic Correlations" by Drs. Leopold Koss and Rana Hoda. I first learned about Leo in the mid-1960s in New Delhi when I was asked to establish a cytopathology laboratory at the All India Institute of Medical Sciences. The late Dr. Ramalingaswami, a friend of Leo's asked me to look at the "red" book-first edition of his classic "Diagnostic Cytology and Its Histopathologic Basis", published in 1961 by Lippincott. Being a trained pathologist, I was impressed by his correlative approach to cytopathology, so very critical for morphologic interpretations. His concepts have been embraced, not only by me, but have become the mantra of cytopathology globally. I had the good fortune to meet Leo a few years later in the US, and he continues to be a mentor and a revered friend. Leo has cytopathology in his DNA; his name is synonymous with cytology. He has shaped the practice of cytopathology globally. He continues to be extremely productive. This one book has been coauthored by Dr. Rana Hoda. I have known Rana for a number of years; she worked here at Penn before moving to New York. Dr. Hoda is extremely talented and sharp. It is a testimony to her accomplishments that Dr. Koss invited her to be a coauthor.

This book summarizes the passion of Leo. He started his cytology career looking at the voided urine specimens obtained from factory workers. True to his doctrine, this work represents Leo's thoughts, concepts, and wisdom in a small colorful crucible of high-quality photomicrographs of cells and their histopathology. One picture is worth a thousand words is evidenced by the use of limited complementary text. Leo is now over 90, I hope and pray that a most enthusiastic reception by the readership of this book shall add many more years to his productive life.

Philadelphia, PA, USA   Prabodh Gupta, MBBS, MD, FIAC

Preface

Technical progress in the identification of cells derived from the urinary bladder and adjacent organs prompted us to restructure an older book "Diagnostic Cytology of The Urinary Tract" published in 1996. This volume is illustrated, for the most part, with photographs of urinary sediment based on current liquid-based techniques.

Besides clinical observations, a fairly large number of laboratory procedures and tests are currently being advocated for detection and follow-up of tumors of the lower urinary tract. The choice of these procedures should be guided by understanding of the principles of the test, always keeping in mind that the specificity and sensitivity of any test are usually reciprocal. A test of great specificity is likely to have low sensitivity and vice versa. The value of the test for an individual patient depends greatly on clinical and pathologic findings, because behavior of urothelial tumors is not always homogeneous or predictable. We hope that this concise volume will be of practical value to cytologists and urologists in the choice of tests, interpretation of results, and hence in the treatment of patients.

Bronx, NY USA   Leopold G. Koss, MD, Doct. HC (multiple)
New York, NY, USA   Rana S. Hoda, MD, FIAC

Acknowledgments

We wish to gratefully acknowledge the assistance of the following colleagues. Dr. Hiroshi Miyamoto of University of Rochester Medical Center for updating the chapter on immunochemistry and other non-cytologic methods of detection of bladder neoplasms;

Ms. Maxine E. Stevenson, senior transcriptionist of New York Presbyterian Hospital for help in preparation of the manuscript; Dr. Prabodh K. Gupta of University of Pennsylvania Health System and Dr. David Wilbur of Massachusetts General Hospital for providing Millipore Filter and SurePath images.

Bronx, NY USA   Leopold G. Koss, MD, Doct. HC (multiple)
New York, NY, USA   Rana S. Hoda, MD, FIAC

Contents

Chapter 1
Introduction

Keywords Urothelium • Hematuria • *Schistosoma hematobium* • Squamous cell carcinoma • Urinalysis • Urine cytology

Historical Note

Examination of urine as a means of diagnosis of human illness has been known since the time of the ancient Egyptians. Badr noted that red urine (hematuria), as evidence of infection with *Schistosoma hematobium* (bilharzia), was recorded in the papyrus of Kahun (1900 B.C.) (Fig. 1.1). The famous Elbers papyrus (1550 B.C.) suggested that hematuria was due to "worms in the belly" (El-Bolkainy). The ancient Egyptians were also aware of the relationship between agricultural activities in the fields irrigated by the river Nile and bloody urine. This relationship was clarified only in 1852 with the discovery of *S. hematobium* by Theodore Bilharz. The relationship of schistosomiasis to bladder cancer was first established by Ferguson in 1911. The mechanism of this association remains unknown.

From the time of Hippocrates into the nineteenth century, the examination of urine was thought to be an important diagnostic procedure. The smell, color, and transparency of the urine and the amount and nature of the sediment, often examined in specially constructed glass containers, was considered to be a guide to diagnosis and treatment of the underlying disorder (Fig. 1.2). There were several sixteenth and seventeenth century paintings of physicians examining urine at the bedside or practicing "uroscopy." Perhaps the epitome of this "science" was a pamphlet published in London in 1637 by Thomas Brian, Member of Parliament, entitled *"The Pisse-prophet or certaine pisse pot lectures. Wherein are newly discovered the old fallacies, deceit, and juggling of the Pisse-pot Science, used by all those (whether Quacks and Empirics, or other methodicall Physicians) who pretend knowledge of Diseases, by the Urine, in giving judgment of the same."*

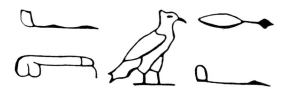

Fig. 1.1 Hematuria, as recorded in the papyrus of Kahun (1900 B.C.), with reference to schistosomiasis (Badr M: Schistosomiasis in Ancient Egypt. In El-Bolkainy, MN and Chu EW Eds: Detection of bladder cancer associated with schistosomiasis. Cairo, Egypt: The National Cancer Institute 1981)

L.G. Koss and R.S. Hoda, *Koss's Cytology of the Urinary Tract with Histopathologic Correlations*, DOI 10.1007/978-1-4614-2056-9_1, © Leopold G. Koss 2012

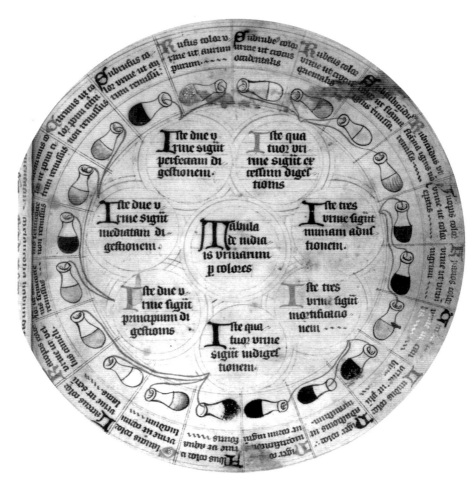

Fig. 1.2 Medieval uroscopy chart used in diagnosis. Note the appearance of glass urinals surrounding the diagnostic options. (Manuscript Ashmole 391 [V], fol. 10r, courtesy of Bodleian Library, Oxford, UK)

In a remarkable article on the subject of uroscopy Fishman (1993) commented on the work of Brian in seventeenth century England. Brian ridiculed the practice of uroscopy, which was often based on examination of urine alone, in the absence of the patient. Samples were often brought to the practioner's office by servants or family members. Brian's pamphlet describes various ruses used by the seventeenth century physicians to obtain from the messengers helpful information about the patient. It is of interest that the vestiges of these fraudulent practices persisted until the early days of the twentieth century. Fishman cited and illustrated a 1911 advertisement by a company in Grand Rapids, Michigan, to establish a diagnosis and prescribe treatment based on analysis of mailed urine samples.

The nineteenth century brought with it major changes in the examination of urine. Besides the progress in organic chemistry that allowed the study of the major organic constituents of urine and their correlation with disease states, microscopic examination of the urinary sediment slowly entered into the medical armamentarium. The ordinary "urinalysis," persisting until today, calls for a casual microscopic examination of unstained urinary sediment for the presence of erythrocytes, leukocytes, and epithelial cells. Staining of the urinary sediment that would have allowed a more detailed examination of the cells was introduced only in the twentieth century. Today, machines capable of automated image analysis of the urinary sediment have replaced the human eye in many laboratories.

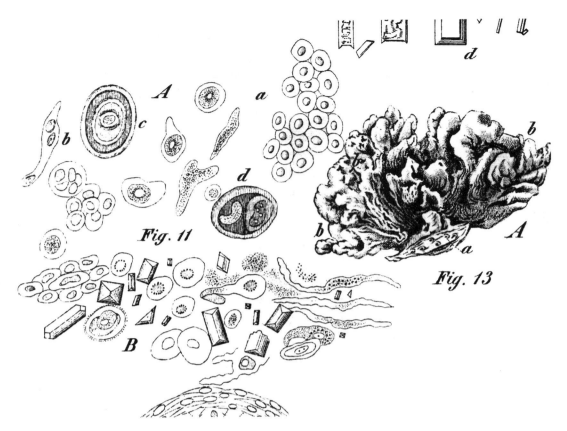

Fig. 1.3 Figure 11 (*left*) from Lambl's 1856 paper, illustrating various cells and crystals observed in the urinary sediment. Figure 13 (*right*) shows "papillary pseudoplasma from the urethra of a girl"-undoubtedly a condyloma accuminatum

Careful microscopic analysis of cells in the urinary sediment began in the middle of the nineteenth century. In 1856 Wilhelm Duschan Lambl (also known as Vilem Dusan Lambl), a Czech physician from Prague, wrote in German a beautifully illustrated article entitled "Ueber Blasenkrebs. Ein Beitrag zur mikroskopischen Diagnostik am Krakenbette" [On cancer of the bladder. A contribution to microscopic diagnosis at bedside], in which he said the following: "The diagnosis of cancer of the bladder by microscopy of the urinary sediment has received no thorough treatment in the available literature— or rather has not been mentioned at all." He then proceeded to describe in considerable detail the cytologic findings in six tumors of the bladder, one uterine carcinoma involving the bladder, one "benign papilloma" of the urethra observed in a girl (presumably a condyloma acuminatum), and two inflammatory conditions serving as controls (Fig. 1.3). Lambl's life story and contributions were described in some detail by two meritorious historians of human cytology, Heinz Grunze and Arthur Spriggs (1986). It is of incidental interest that Lambl's contributions were not limited to bladder cancer. He was immortalized in the name of the parasite *Giardia lamblia*.

Other nineteenth-century observers reported on the diagnostic value of cytology in tumors of the urinary tract. The great British microscopist Beale, who in 1854 published one of the most comprehensive and astute books on the subject of clinical microscopy, subsequently wrote extensively on urinary cytology and in 1864 described cancer cells in the urine. In the same year, a Scottish physician, Sanders, described in Edinburgh Medical Journal a patient in whose urinary sediment fragments of cancerous tissue were observed. Shortly thereafter, in 1869, a British physician, Dickinson, reported

Principal Diagnostic Approach

Needle aspiration

Exfoliative cytology (voided urine, washings, brushings)

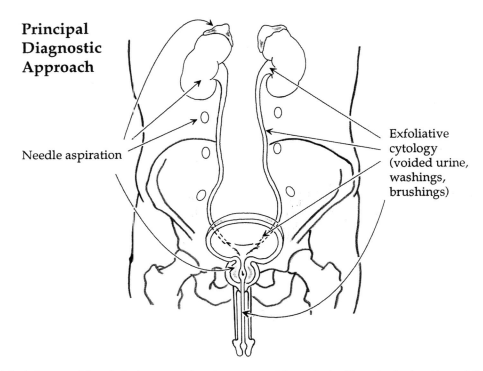

Fig. 1.4 A diagram of the principal organs of the urinary tract and the methods of investigation by either exfoliative or aspiration cytology. (Diagram by Dr. Diane Hamele-Bena, Columbia Presbyterian Hospital, New York, NY). In this book, fine needle aspiration of the kidney is not described (see Koss LG, Melamed MR. Koss's Diagnostic cytology and its histopathologic bases. 5th ed. Philadelphia, PA: Lippincott; 2006. p. 1457–1482)

a similar observation. While there may have been other sporadic reports on this subject that are not known to us, it is noteworthy that in 1892, a New York pathologist, Frank Ferguson, stated at a meeting of the New York Pathological Society that the microscopic examination of histologic sections of paraffin-embedded urinary sediment is one of the most important diagnostic procedures in bladder cancer.

There is no evidence that Ferguson's observations were noted by the medical community: there are no records of cytologic diagnosis of cancer of the lower urinary tract before 1945. In that year Papanicolaou and the urologist, Marshall, reported on the cytologic examination of the urinary sediment in 83 patients. The diagnostic results were reported as 88.8% correct "positive" and 60% correct "negative," thus hardly worthy of note, were it not for the illustrious authors and the fact that the article appeared in the exclusive scientific journal *Science*. In the 1950s, Geoffrey Crabbe, a British cytopathologist, published several papers on the application of voided urine cytology to the surveillance of workers at high risk for bladder cancer who were employed in the dyestuff industries in England, where carcinogenic aromatic amines were produced in open systems. Crabbe's contributions proved to be of seminal value, as they led to a series of observations of workers exposed to a potent bladder carcinogen, paraaminodiphenyl, in the United States. A series of publications by Koss et al. in 1960 1965 and 1969 defined the diagnostic limits and achievements of cytology of voided urine and introduced the concept of *nonpapillary carcinoma* in situ as the principal precursor lesion of invasive cancer of the urinary bladder. These observations have completely modified the approach to the diagnosis and treatment of tumors of the bladder (for further comments see Chap. 5).

The examination of voided urine is an efficient method of diagnosis of some diseases of the lower urinary tract, i.e., bladder, urethra, ureters, and renal pelves. With the passage of time, examination of urine has been supplemented by other methods of securing cell samples. Thus, lavage (washings), brushings, and aspiration biopsy techniques have been applied to these organs. Figure 1.4 summarizes the targets of cytologic diagnosis of organs of interest to urologists.

In this work, we will discuss the fundamental principles underlying the cytologic diagnosis and differential diagnosis of cancer of the lower urinary tract in various types of samples. The various methods of collection and processing of the specimens are described. The use and value of new contemporary approaches to urinary cytology and the diagnosis and monitoring of tumors namely flow cytometry, immunocytochemistry, fluorescence in situ hybridization, and other molecular tests are discussed.

Suggested Readings

1. Adams F. The genuine work of Hippocrates. New York: William Wood; 1886.
2. Badr M. Schistosomiasia in ancient Egypt. In: El-Bolkainy MN, Chu EW, editors. Detection of bladder cancer associated with schistosomiasia. Cairo, Egypt: The National Cancer Institute, Cairo University/Al-Ahram Press; 1981. p. 1–8.
3. Beale LS. The microscope and its application to clinical medicine. London: Highley; 1854.
4. Beale LS. Urine, urinary deposits and calculi and on the treatment of urinary diseases. 2nd ed. London: J. Churchill; 1864.
5. Bilharz T. Ein Beitrag zur elminthographia humana au brieflichen Mittheilungen des Dr. Bilharz in Cairo, nebst Bermerkungen von C.T.V. Siebolt. Z Wissenschaftl Zool. 1852;4:53–76.
6. Brian T. The Pisse-Prophet or certaine pissepot lectures. Wherein are newly discovered the old fallacies, deceit, and juggling of the pisse-pot science, used by all those (whether Quacks and Empiricks, or other methodicall Physicians) who pretend knowledge of Diseases, by the Urine, in giving judgement of the same. London: R. Thrale; 1637
7. Crabbe JGS. Cytological methods of control for bladder tumours of occupational origin. In: Wallace DM, editor. Tumours of the bladder. Edinburgh: Livingstone; 1959. p. 56–76.
8. Crabbe JGS. Cytology of voided urine with special reference to "benign" papilloma and some of the problems encountered in the preparation of the smears. Acta Cytol. 1961;5:233–40.
9. Crabbe JGS, Cresdee WC, Scott TS, Williams MHC. Cytological diagnosis of bladder tumours among dyestuff workers. Br J Ind Med. 1956;13:270–6.
10. Dickinson WH. Portions of cancerous growth passed by the urethra. Tr Path Soc Lond. 1869;20:233–7.
11. Ferguson AR. Associated bilharziasis and primary malignant diseases of the urinary bladder with observations on a series of forty cases. J Pathol Bacteriol. 1911;16:76–94.
12. Ferguson F. The diagnosis of tumors of the bladder by microscopical examination. N.Y. Pathological Society Meeting of April 27, 1892. p. 71–73
13. Fishman D. Pisse-prophets and puritans: Thomas Brian, uroscopy and seventeenth-century English medicine. Pharos. 1993;56:6–11.
14. Grunze H, Spriggs AI. What did Dr. Lambl say in 1856 about cancer cells in urine? Zeiss Inform Oberkochen. 1986;28:44–6.
15. Koss LG, Melamed MR, Kelly RE. Further cytologic and histologic studies of bladder lesions in workers exposed to para-aminodiphenyl. J Natl Cancer Inst. 1969;46:585–95.
16. Koss LG, Melamed MR, Ricci A, et al. Carcinogenesis in the human urinary bladder. Observations after exposure to para-aminodiphenyl. N Engl J Med. 1965;272:767–70.
17. Koss LG, Melamed MR. Koss's diagnostic cytology and its histopathologic bases, Chapter 22. 5th ed. Philadelphia, PA: Lippincott; 2006. p. 738–76.
18. Melamed MR, Koss LG, Ricci A, et al. Cytohistological observations on developing carcinoma of urinary bladder in men. Cancer. 1960;13:67–74.
19. Papanicolaou GN, Marshall VF. Urine sediment smears: A diagnostic procedure in cancers of the urinary tract. Science. 1945;101:519–21.
20. Sanders WK. Cancer of the bladder. Edin Med J. 1864;111:273–4.

Chapter 2
Indication, Collection, and Laboratory Processing of Cytologic Samples

Keywords Indications for urine cytology • Follow up of bladder cancer • Methods of collection • Voided urine • Catheterized urine • Direct sampling techniques • Bladder washings • Bladder barbotage • Direct brushings • Ileal conduit • Retrograde catheterization • Liquid-based preparations • ThinPrep • SurePath • Advantages and disadvantages of various preparations • Laboratory processing techniques for liquid-based preparations • Fixatives for liquid-based preparations • Space-occupying lesions • Occult malignant tumors

Urine is an acellular liquid product of renal excretory function. As liquid passes through the renal tubules, renal pelvis, ureter, urinary bladder, and urethra, it picks up desquamating cells derived from the epithelia of these organs. Inflammatory cells, erythrocytes and macrophages are frequently seen. Voided urine has an acid pH and a high content of urea and other organic components; therefore it is not isotonic. Consequently, urine is not a hospitable medium for desquamated cells, which are often poorly preserved and sometimes difficult to access microscopically.

General

Urinalysis is a standard procedure on all patients. Detecting the presence of albumin, glucose, ketone, bilirubin, occult blood, nitrate, leucocyte esterase, and a superficial analysis of urinary sediment are routine. Machines capable of automated procedures in the assessment of these factors are in wide use and are helpful in the diagnosis and follow-up of a wide variety of diseases. In patients whose lower urinary tract is intact the epithelial sediment is very scanty.

The principal indications for use of cytology in disorders of the lower urinary tract (bladder, urethra, ureters, and renal pelves) are as follows:

1. The diagnosis of high grade urinary cancers, most importantly, flat carcinoma in situ; the cytologic techniques are of a very limited value in the identification of well-differentiated (low grade) papillary tumors.
2. Routinely used in the follow-up of patients with a history of bladder cancer because close monitoring of patients is essential for the early detection of recurrences. The current standard of care consists of cystoscopy and cytology every 3–6 months for the first year and at reduced intervals subsequently.

For the upper urinary tract, cytologic techniques serve to may identify the nature of space-occupying lesions.

L.G. Koss and R.S. Hoda, *Koss's Cytology of the Urinary Tract with Histopathologic Correlations*,
DOI 10.1007/978-1-4614-2056-9_2, © Leopold G. Koss 2012

Methods of Specimen Collection

The principal methods of specimen collection are:

- Voided urine
- Catheterized urine
- Direct sampling techniques

    - Bladder washings or barbotage
    - Cell collection by retrograde catheterization of ureters
    - Direct brushings

The selection of method of specimen collection and processing depends on clinical circumstances and the goal of the examination. Advantages and disadvantages of the various methods are summarized in Table 2.1 and in Chap. 3, Table 3.1.

Voided Urine

This is by far the easiest and the least-expensive method of cytologic investigation of urinary tract. The technique is valuable as preliminary assessment of broad spectrum of abnormalities of the urethra, bladder, ureters, and renal pelves.

Table 2.1 Principle advantages and disadvantages of various cytologic preparatory techniques for urinary specimens

Method	Advantages	Disadvantages
Cytocentrifugation	Simple, large-sized clusters, better-preserved architecture	Air-drying artifact; multiple slides need to be prepared due to cell loss; more unsatisfactory or less than optimal specimens
Membrane Filter	Good morphology	Difficult to prepare, rapid drying makes storage difficult, cells are distorted by pores, cells that are placed in various planes of focus makes screening tedious, background may not be clean, requires fresh specimens as prefixation coagulates proteins that clog the filter; longer screening time
ThinPrep (TP)	Standardized and easy preparation, monolayer, increased cellularity, better preservation, decrease in less-than-optimal specimens, uniform cell distribution, clean background, shorter and easy screening, multiple slides can be prepared, additional cost is offset by improved specimen quality	Some alteration of key nuclear morphologic features and background elements; fragmentation of cell clusters, cell shrinkage; more expensive than conventional preparations
SurePath (SP)	Standardized preparation, excellent cell yield, preservation and morphology, multiple slides can be prepared, slides are stained on the processor	Cells that are in various planes of focus make screening and focusing at high magnification tedious

Collection

Usually the best specimen is the morning's second voiding. Three specimens obtained on 3 consecutive days are diagnostically optimal. Unless the urine is processed without delay, the addition of a fixative is recommended. Small volume of urinary specimen can also be submitted in one of the fixatives described in the liquid-based specimen processing technique section below.

Specimen Fixation

Fresh urine samples that are delivered to the laboratory for processing within 6–12 h of voiding do not require fixation. These specimens should be promptly processed. Specimens fixed in 50% ethanol do not require refrigeration for 24–48 h. Specimens fixed in liquid collection media do not require refrigeration and are described below.

Catheterized Urine

The specimens are collected via a catheter and processed like voided urine as described below.

Direct Sampling techniques

Bladder Washings and Barbotage

This technique may be applied during cystoscopic examination or via a catheter to obtain well-preserved cells from clinically high-risk patients. It is the specimen of choice for DNA ploidy analysis of the urinary epithelium. Bladder washings have significantly better diagnostic yields. The bladder should first be emptied by catheter. Bladder barbotage is then best performed during or prior to cystoscopy by instilling and recovering three to four times 50–100 ml of normal saline or Ringer's solution. The procedure can also be performed through a catheter but is uncomfortable, particularly for male patients, and the results are less satisfactory.

Retrograde Catheterization of Ureters or Renal Pelves

This procedure is used to establish the nature of a space-occupying lesion of ureter or renal pelvis, observed by radiologic techniques. Differential diagnosis of a space-occupying lesion includes a stone, a blood clot, or a tumor. Other rare space-occupying lesions of the renal pelves are inflammatory masses, angiomas, and congenital aberrations of the vascular bed. In the ureters, other causes include a stricture or extraneous pressure.

Another important application of this technique is the localization of an occult malignant tumor diagnosed in voided urine sediment but not found in the bladder. The purpose is to determine whether the tumor can be localized in the left or right kidney or ureter. For urine collection, separate catheters must be used for each side to avoid cross-contamination. Although, the procedure may be tedious to the patient, it is quite efficient in localizing the lesion.

The Direct Brushing Procedure

This procedure is used in the investigation of space-occupying lesions in the ureters or renal pelves. Brushing is performed through a ureteral catheter. The indications are same as listed for retrograde catheterization.

Ileal Bladder Urine

After cystectomy for malignant tumors of the urinary bladder an artificial bladder is often constructed from segments of the small intestine, notably the ileum. Because of the propensity of urothelial tumors to sequentially affect various segments of the lower urinary tract (and sometimes segments of the intestinal tract), the status of these organs must be monitored after treatment. Collection of urine from the ileal bladder serves this purpose well.

Laboratory Processing of Urinary Specimens

Several techniques are available for processing urinary specimens for microscopy including liquid-based preparations (LBP), cytocentrifugation, and membrane filters. Only the two currently available LBP, including ThinPrep [TP (Hologic, Bedford, MA)] or SurePath [SP (BD Diagnostics, Burlington, NC)] will be described in this chapter. Details on semiautomated Bales' Method, cytocentrifugation, and membrane filters preparatory techniques have previously been documented in detail in Koss's Diagnostic Cytology and Its Histologic Bases, by Koss LG and Melamed MR, 5th edition, 2006 and Diagnostic Cytology of the Urinary Tract by Koss LG, 1996. Liquid-based preparations are gaining popularity in the last few years for processing non-gynecologic specimens, particularly, urinary specimens. It is designed to prepare uniform monolayer cells on a glass slide with minimal background blood and cell debris. Table 2.1 lists the various preparatory techniques, their advantages and disadvantages. Liquid-based urinary samples can be collected fresh or in the proprietary liquid preservative media for processing.

Liquid-Based Processing Techniques

Two LBP currently in use include SurePath (SP) and ThinPrep (TP). Both LBP techniques reduce debris and cell clumps and also homogenize the specimen. Due to smaller screening area the slide screening time is reduced and the cleaner background makes it easier to determine whether the cells are normal or abnormal. Immediate liquid fixation prevents air-drying. Despite the difference in preparatory techniques, both TP and SP are similar in morphologic appearance. Technical details for the two LBP are provided in Figs. 2.1 and 2.2 and Tables 2.2, 2.3, and 2.4 outline technical, general cytologic, and specific cellular features for the LBP.

SurePath

Principle

The principle of SP is density gradient-based cell enrichment process. It is a semi-automated technique. Specimen is processed on the PrepStain processor.

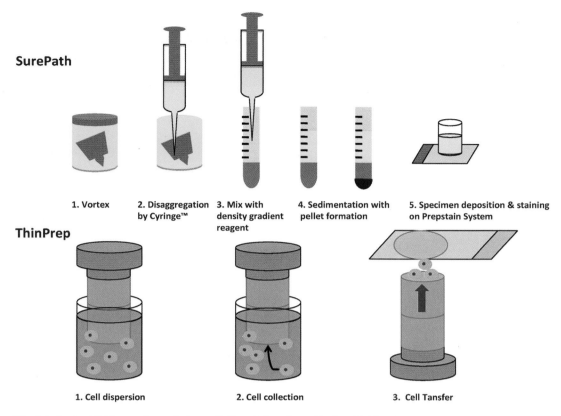

SurePath

1. Vortex   2. Disaggregation   3. Mix with   4. Sedimentation with   5. Specimen deposition & staining
              by Cyringe™   density gradient   pellet formation   on Prepstain System
                                reagent

ThinPrep

1. Cell dispersion   2. Cell collection   3. Cell Tansfer

Fig. 2.1 SurePath™ Processing technique: (1) Sample is collected in CytoRich®-(ethanol-based SP preservative fluid) filled collection vial and vortexed; (2) A SP proprietary device, CyRinge, is inserted into the collection vial to disaggregate larger cell fragments; (3) The CyRinge is then inverted over a labeled 15-ml centrifuge tube filled with 4 ml of SP density gradient reagent, a polysaccharide solution that acts to trap small particulates and debris. The samples flow through the drainage tube on the CyRinge onto the density gradient; (4) Specimen is transferred to a sedimentation tube and centrifuged to form a cell pellet, which is resuspended and the sedimentation is repeated; (5) Sample processing is completed using the PrepStain™ slide processor, where a robotic arm transfers the fluid to a settling chamber, which sits atop a modified poly-L-lysine-coated glass slide. Robotic arm then stains the slides on the PrepStain™. ThinPrep™ Processing technique: (1) Cell dispersion. A cylinder with a polycarbonate thin filter attached to one end is introduced into the specimen vial and gently rotated creating a current that disaggregates mucus, blood, and other debris; breaks up large cell clusters; and mixes and homogenizes the cell suspension; (2) Cell Collection: A gentle vacuum is applied to the cylinder that causes most of the broken erythrocytes and debris to pass through the filter pores, while the cells adhere to the filter. The instrument monitors cell density across the filter and the flow rate decreases when cells are evenly distributed on the filter with minimal overlap; (3) Cell Transfer: The cylinder moves out of the specimen and is lightly pressed against a positively charged slide. A slightly positive air pressure is applied to transfer the cells to the slide. The slide is immediately dropped into 95% ethanol fixative. Slide is removed from the processor and may be stained either manually or by an automatic stainer (modified from: Cibas ES and Ducatman BS. Liquid-based preparation methods. In Cytology. Diagnostic Principles and Clinical Correlations. 3rd ed., Saunders, Philadelphia, PA, 2009, p. 5. Drawing by Raza Hoda, Columbia University College of Physicians and Surgeons, New York, NY)

Specimen Collection and Fixation

Non-gynecologic specimens are collected in one of the following: CytoRich® Preservative Fluid (an ethanol-based medium, which also lyses blood), in 50% alcohol, or as fresh, unfixed specimens. Specimen is labeled and transported to the cytology laboratory.

Fig. 2.2 ThinPrep (TP) and SurePath (SP) Slides: For the TP slide, the circle where the cytologic material is deposited has a diameter of 20 mm. The specimen collection preservative medium is methanol based. For SP slide, the diameter of the circle is 13 mm, and the specimen collection preservative medium is ethanol based

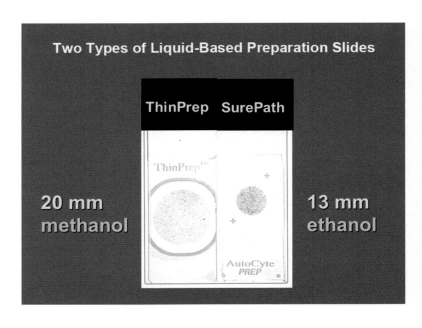

Table 2.2 Technical differences between LBP preparations

Features	ThinPrep	SurePath
Cost	Expensive	Less expensive
Sample collection	Uniform	Uniform
Sample transfer	Entire	Entire
Fixation	Immediate	Immediate
Transport	Easy	Easy
Slide preparation	Fully automated	Partial automation
Slide evaluation	Easier	Easy
Cells deposition	Well defined 20-mm-diameter area	Well defined 13-mm-diameter area
Cell preservation	Good	Good
Obscuring factors	None	None
Air-drying	None	None
Screening time	Reduced	Reduced
Reproducibility	Yes	Yes
Ancillary studies	Possible	Possible

Table 2.3 General cytologic features on LBP preparations

Features	ThinPrep	SurePath
Quality	Enhanced	Enhanced
Background		
Clean	Yes	Yes
RBCs	Reduced	More reduced
Neutrophils	Reduced	Reduced
Necrosis	Clumped	Clumped
Cellularity	Lower	Higher
Cell distribution	Uniform, one plane of focus	Uniform, thick, different planes of focus
Cell size	Smaller	Small
Architecture	Less well-preserved	Better preserved
Cytomorphology	Preserved	Preserved
Extracellular material		
Quantity	Reduced	Less reduced
Appearance	Altered	Less altered

Table 2.4 Specific cellular features of LBP preparations

Features	ThinPrep	SurePath
Architecture		
Fragmentation	Present ++	Present +
Monolayer cells	+	–
Cell clusters	Present, 3D	Present, thick, 3D
	Flat, smaller	>Depth of focus
	Cohesive	Cohesive
	Minimal overlap	More overlap
Flattening	More	Less
Cellular morphology		
Shape	More rounded	Rounded/elongated
Nucleus		
Detail	Enhanced	Enhanced
Nucleoli	More prominent	Preserved
Inclusions	Less apparent	Preserved
Cytoplasm		
Detail	May be denser	May be denser
Shape	Retained	Retained
Elements[a]	Preserved	Preserved

+ present, – not present

[a] Cytoplasmic elements include: vacuolations, pigment, PMNs

Slides

Pre-coated slides are provided by the company and are marked with a 13-mm-diameter circle. The slides can also be freshly prepared in the laboratory for use for 48 h. The slides are coated with a modified poly-L-lysine and air-dried. These positively charged slides allow diagnostic cells to settle out of solution and adhere to the surface.

Processing

1. Mix entire specimen to resuspend cellular material. In large-volume samples, pour off one or two aliquots into 50-ml centrifuge tubes, cap securely, and centrifuge for 10 min at 1,800 rpm to concentrate the specimen.
2. Decant off the supernatant and add 10 ml of distilled water.
3. Vortex the cell button to form a homogeneous cell slurry. Transfer 5–10 drops of the cell slurry to 10 ml of CytoRich® Red Preservative Fluid and mix to an even cell suspension. Sample may also be received in a vial with CytoRich collection fluid.
4. Specimen collection vials are vortexed. CytoRich fluid lyses most of the red blood cells.
5. A SurePath proprietary device, CyRinge®, is inserted into the collection vial to disaggregate larger cell fragments. CyRinge is a syringe-like device consisting of a double-layered mesh screen with 18-gauge holes in its base and a drainage tube extending from its top.
6. The CyRinge is then inverted over a labeled 15-ml centrifuge tube filled with 4 ml of SurePath density gradient reagent, a polysaccharide solution that acts to trap small particulates and debris. The samples flow through the drainage tube on the CyRinge onto the density gradient reagent.
7. Specimen is transferred to a sedimentation tube to concentrate the cellular components of the specimen by centrifuging the specimen on the Hettich Centrifuge $600 \times g$ for 10 min. A cell pellet is formed, which is resuspended and the sedimentation is repeated.

8. Load the centrifuge racks onto the PrepStain Processor and run Program 2 for Non-GYN specimens. A robotic arm transfers the fluid to a settling chamber, which sits atop a modified poly-L-lysine-coated glass slide. Robotic arm then delivers sequential stains to each settling chamber to stain the specimen. The result is a 13-mm circular smear. PrepStain System processes and stains up to 48 specimens per run.

ThinPrep

Principle

ThinPrep preparation is a filter-based cell concentration technique. TP-2000 processor is a semiautomated device, which processes one specimen at a time. A newer version, TP-5000, is a fully automated bench-top instrument that processes specimens in batches of 20. Multiple preparations can be made from a single vial.

Specimen Collection and Fixation

Sample is collected by the clinician in one of the following: CytoLyte® solution (methanol-based fixative, which is both hemolytic and mucolytic), in saline, or as fresh, unfixed specimens. Specimen is labeled and transported to the cytology laboratory.

Slides

The microscopic slides are provided by the company and are marked with a 20-mm diameter circle.

Steps in Preparation

Urine is first centrifuged at 1,500 rpm and cell pellet is then resuspended in 30 ml of Cytolyte and again centrifuged. Two to three drops of the cell pellet are transferred to PreservCyt (methanol-based preservative solution). The vial and a labeled slide are placed into the ThinPrep processor. Preparatory steps include specimen dispersion, collection, transfer, and staining.

(a) *Dispersion*. A disposable cylinder with a polycarbonate filter attached to one end is introduced into the vial. The pore size of the filter is 5.5 µm (pore size for Pap test specimen is 8 µm). The instrument is rotated creating a current that disaggregates blood, mucus, and other debris and breaks up large cell clusters, mixes and homogenizes the cell suspension.

(b) *Collection*. A gentle vacuum is applied to the cylinder, which aspirates the cell suspension through the filter. Most of the broken red blood cells and debris is allowed to pass through while the diagnostic cells attach to the external surface of the filter. The instrument monitors cell density across the filter and the flow rate decreases when cells are evenly distributed on the filter with minimal overlap.

(c) *Transfer*. the cylinder moves out of the specimen, is inverted 180°, gently pressed against a positively charged slide and with slight positive pressure transfers the cells (~70,000) to the glass slide. The result is a 20-mm circular smear with even distribution of cells and minimal overlap.

The slide is immediately dropped into 95% ethanol fixative. Preparation time ranges between 30 and 90 s depending on cell concentration.

(d) *Staining*. Papanicolaou staining is either performed manually or in an automatic stainer. The staining process takes 30 min. Papanicolaou stain of fixed samples offers the best option of judging the fine details of cell structure. All illustrations in this book are stained with this method.

Residual LBP Specimen

The shelf life of the residual specimen for SP and TP is 3 weeks and 3 months, respectively, at room temperature. Residual specimen can be used for immunochemistry, molecular tests such as UroVysion (Chap. 7) or processed as a cell block. Cellient (Hologic, Bedford, MA) is a new automated cell block machine based on centrifugation and filtration and can capture cells from a low cellularity specimen such as a urinary specimen.

Liquid-based preparations (LBP) are increasingly being used for urinary cytology. The LBP have several advantages over the conventional preparatory techniques including standardized preparation, uniform (monolayered) cell distribution, lack of obscuring elements, better cell preservation with enhanced nuclear detail due to immediate wet fixation, and decreased rate of unsatisfactory specimens. These features of LBP have resulted in increased diagnostic accuracy compared to conventional preparations.

Residual material from LBP fixed in the proprietary fixatives may also be used for ancillary studies such as immunocytochemistry and fluorescence in situ hybridization.

Suggested Readings

1. Ajit D, Dighe SB, Desai SB. Cytology of ileal conduit urine in bladder cancer patients: diagnostic utility and pitfalls. Acta Cytol. 2006;50:70–3.
2. Bales CE. A semiautomated method for preparation of urine sediment for cytologic evaluation. Acta Cytol. 1981;25:323–6.
3. Cibas ES. Cervical and vaginal cytology: processing of liquid-based preparations. In: Cytology: diagnostic principles and clinical correlates. 3rd ed. Philadelphia, PA: Saunders Elsevier; 2009. p. 3–5.
4. Elsheikh TM, Kirkpatrick JL, Wu HH. Comparison of ThinPrep and cytospin preparations in the evaluation of exfoliative cytology specimens. Cancer. 2006;108:144–9.
5. Hoda RS. Non-gynecologic cytology on liquid-based preparations: a morphologic review of facts and artifacts. Diagn Cytopathol. 2007;35:621–34. Review.
6. Hundley AF, Maygarden S, Wu JM, et al. Adequacy of urine cytology specimens: an assessment of collection techniques. Int Urogynecol J. 2007;18:997–1001.
7. Koss LG, Melamed MR. The lower urinary tract in the absence of cancer. In: Koss LG, Melamed MR, editors. Koss's Diagnostic Cytology and its Histopathologic Bases. 5th ed. Philadelphia, PA: Lippincott Williams & Wilkins; 2006. p. 738–76.
8. Koss LG. Indications, collection, and laboratory processing in cytologic samples. In: Diagnostic Cytology of the Urinary Tract. Philadelphia, PA: Lippincott-Raven; 1996. p. 3–15.
9. Koss LG, Deitch D, Ramanathan R, et al. Diagnostic value of cytology of voided urine. Acta Cytol. 1985; 29:810–6.
10. Laucirica R, Bentz JS, Souers RJ, et al. Do liquid-based preparations of urinary cytology perform differently than classically prepared cases? Observations from the College of American Pathologists Interlaboratory Comparison Program in Nongynecologic Cytology. Arch Pathol Lab Med. 2010;134:19–22.
11. Laudadio J, Keane TE, Reeves HM, et al. Fluorescence in situ hybridization for detecting transitional cell carcinoma: implications for clinical practice. BJU Int. 2005;96:1280–5.
12. Luthra UK, Dey P, George J, et al. Comparison of ThinPrep and conventional preparations: urine cytology evaluation. Diagn Cytopathol. 1999;21:364–6.

13. Michael CW, McConnel J, Pecott J. Comparison of ThinPrep and TriPath PREP liquid-based preparations in nong-
    ynecologic specimens: a pilot study. Diagn Cytopathol. 2001;25:177–84.
14. Moonen PM, Peelen P, Kiemeney LA, et al. Quantitative cytology on bladder wash versus voided urine: a compari-
    son of results. Eur Urol. 2006;49:1044–9.
15. Nassar H, Ali-Fehmi R, Madan S. Use of ThinPrep monolayer technique and cytospin preparation in urine cytol-
    ogy: a comparative analysis. Diagn Cytopathol. 2003;28:115–8.
16. Nagai S, Murase Y, Yokoyama M, et al. Comparison of urine cytology between the ileal conduit and Indiana pouch.
    Acta Cytol. 2000;44:748–51.
17. Nasuti JF, Tam D, Gupta PK. Diagnostic value of liquid-based (ThinPrep) preparations in nongynecologic cases.
    Diagn Cytopathol. 2001;24:137–41.
18. Piaton E, Faÿnel J, Hutin K, et al. Conventional liquid-based techniques versus Cytyc ThinPrep® processing of
    urinary samples: a qualitative approach. BMC Clin Pathol. 2005;5:9.
19. Raistrick J, Shambayati B, Dunsmuir W. Collection fluid helps preservation in voided urine cytology. Cytopathology.
    2008;19:111–7.
20. Rowe LR, Marshall J, Bentz JS. PrepMate automated processor: comparison of automated and manual methods of
    liquid-based gynecologic sample preparation. Diagn Cytopathol. 2002;27:312–5.
21. Sng KK, Nga ME, Tan SY, et al. Analysis of urine cytology tests in 120 paired cases. Acta Cytol. 2007;51:782–7.
22. Voss JS, Kipp BR, Krueger AK, et al. Changes in specimen preparation method may impact urine cytologic evalu-
    ation. Am J Clin Pathol. 2008;130:428–33.
23. Watarai Y, Satoh H, Matubara M, et al. Evaluation of thin-layer methods in urine cytology. Cytopathology.
    2001;12:306–13.
24. Zardawi IM, Duncan J. Evaluation of a centrifuge method and thin-layer preparation in urine cytology. Acta Cytol.
    2003;47:1038–42.

Chapter 3
The Cellular and Acellular Components
of the Urinary Sediment

Keywords Normal urothelium • Anatomy of lower urinary tract • Histology of bladder • Trigone • Urine–blood barrier • Superficial urothelial cells • Umbrella cells • Multinucleated umbrella cells • Foreign body giant cells • Langhan's giant cells • Endomitosis • Ultrastructure of umbrella cells • Plaques • Asymmetric Unit Membrane • Uroplakins • Scanning electron microscopy • Embryonal intestinal tract • Variants of urothelium • von Brunn's nests • Parabasal cells • Intermediate cells • Basal cells • Deeper urothelial cells • Instrumentation • Clusters • Liquid-based preparations • Bladder wash • Cytokeratin 20 • Cystitis cystica • Cystitis glandularis • Squamous epithelium • Squamous cells • Pseudomembranous trigonitis • Mucus-producing epithelium • Paneth cells • Bladder extrophy • Adenocarcinoma • Mitosis • Chromatin condensation • Blood cells • Intestinal type cells • Eosinophiluria • Macrophages • Lymphocytes • Renal tubular cells • Prostatic cells • Seminal vesicle cells • Erythrocytes • Leukocytes • Polymorphonuclear leukocytes • Noncellular components • Crystals • Contaminants • Renal casts

Normal Lower Urinary Tract

Urine is a toxic substance produced by the kidney and eliminated from the body by a series of hollow organs of the lower urinary tract, consisting of renal pelves, ureters, bladder, and urethra. Each organ of the lower urinary tract is composed of three layers of tissues: the epithelium, lining the lumen, resting on a layer of connective tissue or the lamina propria, and muscular layers that vary in thickness from organ to organ. These organs are separated from the abdominal cavity by a serosa composed of mesothelial cells, capillary vessels, and loose connective tissue.

The urine, a toxic fluid, is confined to the lumina of the excretory system. There exists, therefore a protection mechanism or a *urine–blood barrier*. The exact role of the component tissues of the lower urinary tract in the effectiveness of the barrier has not been fully determined, but it is likely that the urothelium (previously known as transitional epithelium) plays a major role in this regard.

Anatomy (See Fig. 1.4)

The urine is excreted from the renal tubules into reservoirs, known as renal pelves, roughly triangular, funnel-like structures. The broad end of each renal pelvis encompasses the renal papillae containing terminal tubules, and the narrow end transits into the ureter. Each of the ureters is a relatively rigid

L.G. Koss and R.S. Hoda, *Koss's Cytology of the Urinary Tract with Histopathologic Correlations,*
DOI 10.1007/978-1-4614-2056-9_3, © Leopold G. Koss 2012

tube, measuring about 25 cm in length, its lower end opening into the posterior part of the trigone of the urinary bladder.

The urinary bladder, when empty, is a fist-size hollow organ, next to the prostate in men and on the anterior wall of the vagina in women. The lumen of the bladder is conveniently divided into several areas of segments. The best defined is the floor of the bladder, or the trigone, an approximately triangular structure with an anterior apex pointing towards the urethra. The ureters enter into the bladder in the posterior aspect of the trigone. The remainder of the bladder is divided into an anterior, lateral, and posterior walls. The apex of the bladder or the dome harbors the vestiges of the urachus or the omphalomesenteric duct, connecting the embryonal bladder with the umbilicus. The urine produced by embryonal kidney is excreted into the amniotic fluid. The urine accumulating in the bladder exits through the urethra, a very short organ in women but a long one in men, traversing the entire length of the penis.

The urothelium characteristic of the organs of the lower urinary tract will be described in detail below. The muscular layer, composed of smooth muscle, is thin in the renal pelves and thick in the ureters, accounting for the relative rigidity of the organ.

Normal Urothelium (Transitional Epithelium) and Its Cells

Histology and Ultrastructure

In histologic sections, the normal epithelium lining the human urinary bladder, ureters, and renal pelves is composed of seven to eight layers of cells, provided with a unique superficial layer (Fig. 3.1). The number of cell layers appears to be constant in the ureter but is highly variable in the urinary bladder, depending on the state of dilation or contraction of this organ: fewer cell layers are visible in a dilated bladder than in a contracted bladder (Fig. 3.2a, b). The variability in the number of cell layers is accounted for by a presumed mechanism of cell movements. It is assumed but not proven that the epithelial cells are capable of "sliding" against each other, thus adjusting to the volume requirements without breaking the continuity of the urine–blood barrier.

Another mechanism of epithelial movement was proposed by Petry and Amon (1966). These authors suggested that all epithelial cells, including umbrella cells, are anchored on the basement membrane and thus can adapt to the changing volume of urine without disruption of epithelial continuity. We were unable to confirm the existence of such cytoplasmic extensions in the rat urothelium.

An important feature of the urothelium is the presence of a superficial layer composed of very large, often multinucleated cells that may measure from 20 to 50 μm in diameter. The superficial cells are also known as "umbrella cells" because each one of them extends over several smaller cells of the underlying layer in umbrella-like fashion (see Fig. 3.2a, b). The umbrella cells are provided with

Fig. 3.1 Normal human urothelium (distended bladder). Note the six to seven layers of epithelial cells and the presence of the very large superficial cells (umbrella cells) on the surface. Small capillary vessels are present immediately beneath the epithelium in the lamina propria [H&E ×20 objective]

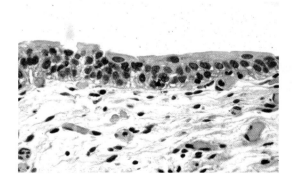

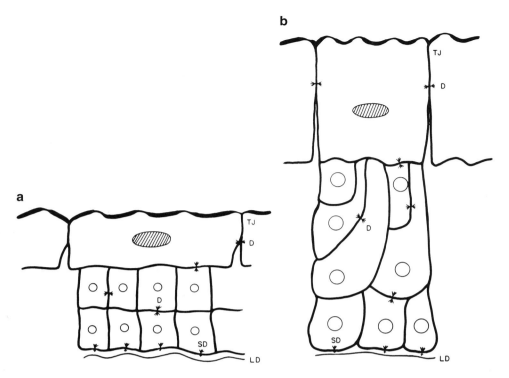

Fig. 3.2 Schematic drawing of the structure of the urothelium in a dilated (**a**) and contracted (**b**) bladder. The cells are bound to each other by desmosomes; the epithelium is bound to the lamina densa (LD) of the basement membrane by hemidesmosomes. Then superficial umbrella cells are bound to each other by tight junctions (TJ). The surface of the umbrella cells is lined by plaques of the asymmetric unit membrane (see also Fig. 3.3). The nuclei of the umbrella cells are larger than those of the deeper cell layers and may be multiple

either single large or multiple smaller nuclei. In some of them the number of nuclei may reach 50. The mechanism of nuclear multiplication is unknown.

The cells of the deeper layers of the urothelium resemble parabasal cells from the deeper layers of the squamous epithelium: they measure from 7 to 10 μm in diameter that increases towards the surface, and are bound to each other by numerous solid cell junctions, the desmosomes. Their nuclei are single, spherical, and open or vesicular. The basal layer of the epithelium, composed of the smallest cells, is bound to the lamina densa of the basement membrane by specialized structures known as hemidesmosomes.

It is of note that there are also immunologic differences between the deeper layers of the urothelium and the superficial umbrella cell layer. Perhaps the most important difference is the expression of keratin 20, which is normally limited to umbrella cells. It has been observed that the expression of this keratin occurring in smaller deeper cells is associated with malignant tumors; an abbreviation of potential diagnostic value (see Chaps. 6 and 7).

Ultrastructure of the Umbrella Cells

The umbrella cells lining the lumen of the organ are bound to each other by tight junctions (Fig. 3.3a), cell devices preventing the seepage of urine across the epithelium. The surface membrane of the urothelial cells has unique ultrastructural characteristics. The principal feature of the membrane are

Fig. 3.3 (A) Electron
microscopic structure of
normal human urothelium.
The two adjacent superficial
cells are bound by a tight
junction (TJ). Numerous
oblong vesicles (V) may be
noted. The angulated surface
reflects the presence of the
asymmetric unit membrane
shown in *inset*. [(**a**) approx.
×24,000; *inset* approx.
×150,000]. (**b**) Scanning
electron micrograph of
superficial urothelial cells in
a distended human bladder.
The surface is covered by
uniform, stubby microridges
(approx. ×5,000)

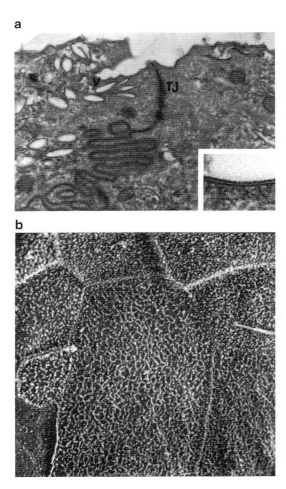

the rigid segments known as *plaques*. The plaques are composed of two electron opaque layers, with an electron-lucent layer sandwiched in between. Because of the unequal thickness of the electron opaque layers this membrane is known as the *asymmetric unit membrane* (AUM) (Fig. 3.3a, inset). The asymmetric unit membrane is formed in the Golgi apparatus of the superficial cells and is packaged in the form of oblong vesicles that travel to the surface, replacing the worn or damaged membrane. In contracted bladder the AUM is stored in the form of invaginations or canals, leading from the surface to depth of the cell. In dilated bladder the canals either disappear or become very shallow, the AUM being used to form the surface of the umbrella cells. Structural proteins known as *uroplakins* are the principal components of the plaques. It is of interest that cultured normal human urothelial cells retain the ability to form AUM.

The plaques are separated from each other by short segments of ordinary, flexible cell membrane that does not have any specific morphologic features, but is characterized by a specific glycoprotein. The apparent role of these segments is to confer flexibility to the plaques so that the superficial cells can adapt to the changing volume of the organ. This is particularly important in reference to the urinary bladder, which may be either distended or contracted depending on the volume of urine. In distended bladder studied by scanning electron microscopy, the umbrella cells are rather flat and their surface is characterized by ridges formed by AUM (Fig. 3.3b). In contracted bladder the umbrella cells are more cuboidal in shape.

Variants of Normal Urothelium

Careful mapping studies of normal urinary bladder obtained at autopsies of people dying of unrelated causes have shown that several epithelial variants may be observed in the lower urinary tract, reflecting in part its origin in the cloaca, i.e., the embryonal intestinal tract. The most common variants are the nests of von Brunn (commonly known as Brunn's nests) and cystitis cystica and glandularis (Fig. 3.4a, b). Brunn's nests are buttonlike dips of urothelium into the lamina propria. The nests are either solid, composed of urothelial cells, or may show small central cysts that may be lined by mucus-producing columnar glandular cells. The center of the cystic nests may contain mucus. The frequency of distribution and the location of Brunn's nests in 61 bladders from males and 39 bladders from females are shown in Fig. 3.4c, d.

Cystitis cystica and glandularis are the terms attached to cystic structures lined by cuboidal or columnar mucus-producing cells. The cysts may be small, limited to lamina propria, or quite large, sometimes involving the epithelium, the lamina propria, and even the muscularis of the bladder (Fig. 3.4a, b). Contrary to the name attached to them, the cysts are not of inflammatory origin but represent a congenital variant of the epithelium. The distribution of cystitis cystica in the normal bladder is shown in Fig. 3.4c, d. This variant is most commonly observed in the area of the trigone.

The presence of *squamous epithelium of vaginal type* in the trigone of the bladder is yet another epithelial variant, observed mainly in women and rarely in men (Fig. 3.5a, b). The term "pseudomembranous trigonitis" has been sometimes applied to this entity although there is no evidence whatever that the squamous epithelium is related to an inflammatory process. It appears likely that the squamous epithelium in women follows the hormonal cyclic changes of the vaginal epithelium. It is not known why squamous epithelium may be rarely observed in the trigone of men.

Areas of *mucus-producing epithelium*, often resembling the epithelium of the small or large bowel, may also line segments of bladder surface, replacing the urothelium (Fig. 3.5c, d). In such epithelial areas specialized enteric cells, such as Paneth cells, may be observed. Exceptionally, ciliated columnar epithelium may be observed.

The urothelial variants have no pathologic significance in normal individuals with the exception of cystitis cystica composed of large cysts that may be symptomatic because of their volume. However, in tumors of the urothelium, especially carcinomas, these variants may be represented either as a subsidiary or as the dominant feature of these tumors. In bladder extrophy the presence of intestinal type of epithelium may predispose to adenocarcinomas (see Chap. 6).

Cells Derived from Normal Urothelium

In cytologic preparations there are two principal characteristics of cells derived from normal urothelium that set them apart from other epithelial structures:

1. *The marked variability in the size and structure of the component cells reflecting the differences between the superficial umbrella cells and cells derived from the deeper layers.*
2. *The tendency of these cells to desquamate in clusters. These features are directly related to the structure of the urothelium described above* (Fig. 3.6a–d).

Superficial (Umbrella) Cells

Regardless of the type of sample and collection technique used, the superficial urothelial cells are a common component of the urine sediment. In desquamated samples the umbrella cells are large cells,

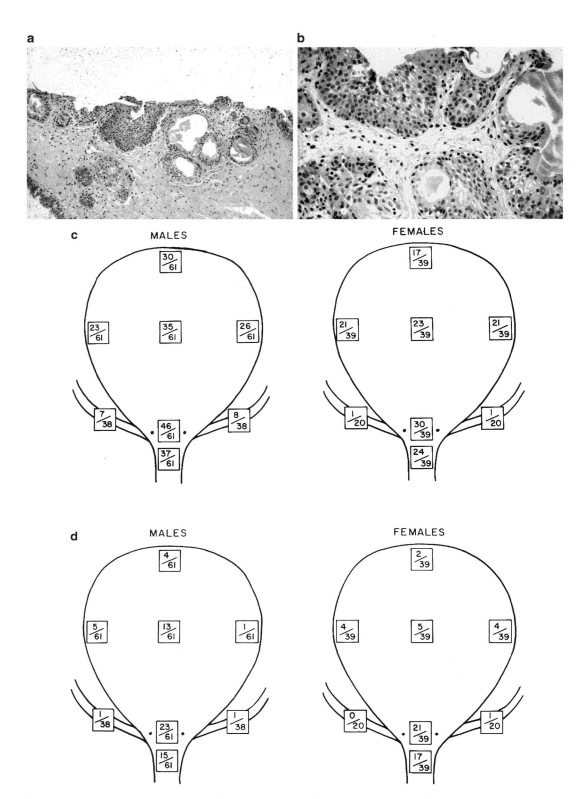

Fig. 3.4 (**a**) Brunn's nests and a focus of "cystitis glandularis." Note the nests of urothelial cells in the lamina propria (H&E ×10); (**b**) One open focus of cystitis glandularis is shown. The latter structure is lined by mucus-producing columnar cells; the lumen is filled with mucus (H&E ×20); (**c, d**) Diagrams showing the frequency and sites of occurrence of these two variants of the urothelium in 61 males and 39 females with normal bladders

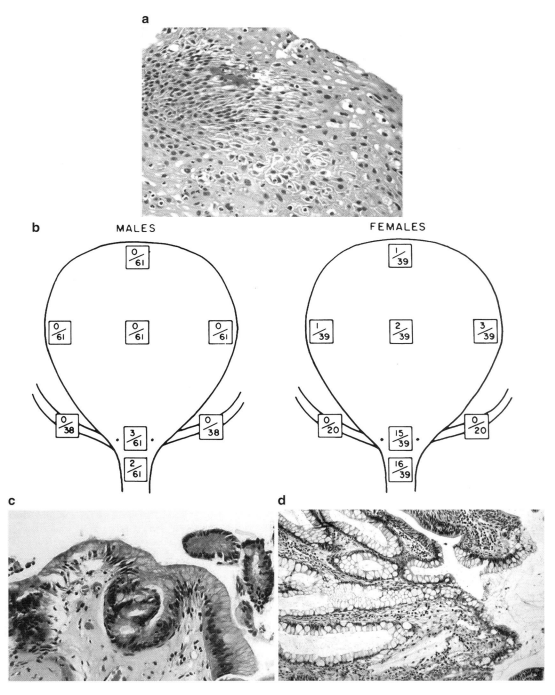

Fig. 3.5 (**a**) An area of squamous epithelium of vaginal type in the bladder trigone of a young woman (H&E ×10); (**b**) A diagram showing the distribution of this variant in 61 males and 39 females: this variant is much more common in the trigone area of women than in men; (**c**) Mucus-producing epithelium of colonic type (intestinal metaplasia) may occur in bladder of otherwise normal people (H&E ×20); (**d**) Mucus-producing epithelium of colonic type in an extrophic bladder. A malignant transformation of this type of epithelium may occur, resulting in carcinomas of intestinal types (H&E ×20)

a   b

c   d

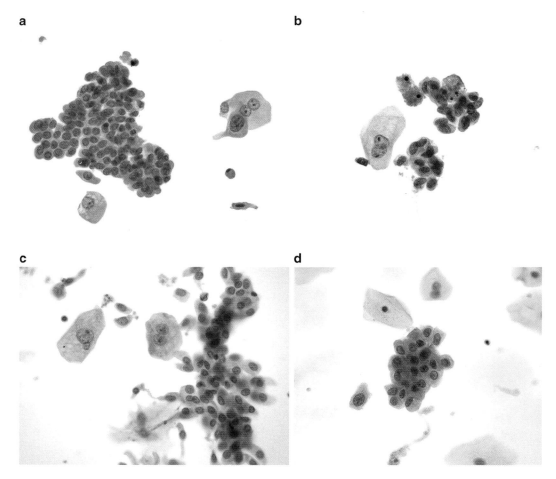

Fig. 3.6 (**a**) Bladder washings and (**b**) catheterized urine on ThinPrep showing two types of urothelial cells, large and small, in the same field. The larger cells are the superficial umbrella cells. The smaller cells are derived from the deeper layers of the urothelium and often desquamate in clusters. Note the angulated thick membrane of the superficial cell and the large nucleus with chromocenter (**a**, **b**, TP ×60); (**c**) Bladder washings and (**d**) voided urine on SurePath showing two types of urothelial cells, large and small in the same field. Note that the features are similar to those seen in TP (**c**, **d**, SP ×60)

somewhat similar in size to superficial squamous cells, but often larger. The cytoplasm often has one flat surface. The nuclei can either be single or multiple, of variable sizes with occasional small nucleoli (Fig. 3.7a–f). To the inexperienced, nuclear features of umbrella cells may suggest the presence of an abnormality or even a malignant process.

The umbrella cells with a single nucleus are more common in voided urine. They are large, measuring 20–30 μm in diameter, and spherical or slightly ovoid in configuration. The single nuclei are large, round with regular finely granular chromatin, sharply demarcated nuclear membrane, and, as mentioned before, small nucleoli may be observed (Fig. 3.7c, d). Binucleated cells are also seen common. Such cells are often larger than the mononucleated umbrella cells and the nuclei are somewhat smaller (Fig. 3.7e, f). The nuclei are still smaller in multinucleated cells but their fundamental structure remains the same. The number of nuclei is variable and may reach 40 or 50, particularly in umbrella cells derived from the ureter (Fig. 3.7g–i).

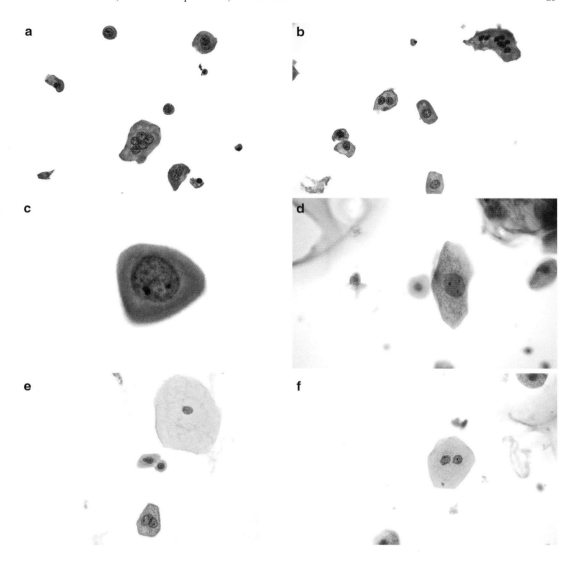

Fig. 3.7 (**a**, **b**) Voided urine: Various types of umbrella including multinucleated, binucleated, and mononucleated in ThinPrep (×40); (**c**, **d**) Voided urine: Umbrella cells with single nuclei. Note small single or multiple nucleoli, finely granular ("salt and pepper" appearance) chromatin and thick, sharply demarcated cell membrane on cell surface (**c**, TP and **d**, SP ×60); (**e**, **f**) Voided urine: Binucleated umbrella cells in SurePath. Note the single nuclei and small nucleoli (×40); (**g**) Large multinucleated umbrella cell in catheterized urine. The nuclei are very large (compare with the benign intermediate cell nuclei in the field) and contain multiple small nucleoli against a background of fine granular chromatin (TP ×60); (**h**) Umbrella cell with numerous small nuclei of variable sizes (*right*) overlying a cell with two nuclei (*top left*). Note large cytoplasmic vacuoles with some containing amorphous material and the sharply demarcated cell membrane (TP ×60). Umbrella cells can be large, forming true giant cells; (**i**) Multinucleated umbrella cells in retrograde catheterization showing numerous small, degenerated, and pyknotic nuclei of variable sizes, mimicking hyperchromasia (TP ×60)

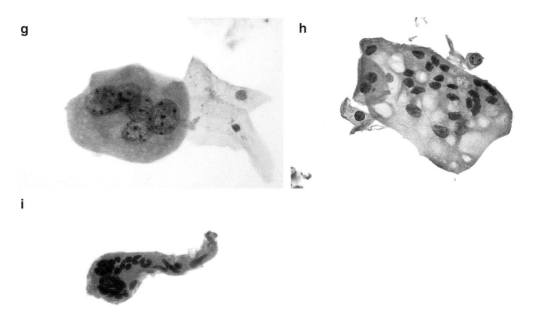

Fig. 3.7 (continued)

The mechanism of formation of the multinucleated umbrella cells is not clear. Cell fusion that accounts for the formation of foreign body giant cells and Langhans' giant cells from epithelioid cells or immobilized small macrophages is extremely unlikely to occur in the urothelium. Hence the best explanation for the occurrence of these cells is endomitosis, a nuclear division taking place without cytoplasmic division. The functional role of the multinucleated cells also remains a mystery. It is not known at this time whether these cells play a role in the formation of the urine–blood barrier. A thin layer of mucus may occasionally be found on the surface of the umbrella cells.

Cells Originating from the Deeper Layers of the Urothelium

The intermediate and basal cells comprise this group of cells (Fig. 3.8a–e). Such cells usually desquamate in clusters. Single small urothelial cells are observed, usually in the presence of an inflammatory process with destruction of the superficial layer, or when removed by an instrument from their natural setting.

Intermediate cells resemble parabasal squamous cells in size and configuration. These cells are often spherical or round and may also occur singly. The cytoplasm of the individual cells is usually scanty and basophilic; it surrounds spherical nuclei that are usually bland and contain one, rarely two, chromocenters.

The basal cells are the deeper cells and are the smallest. The clusters of the deeper cells may be tightly packed and assume a spherical "papillary" configuration with sharp borders. Such clusters are often misinterpreted as reflecting papillary tumors (see Chaps. 4 and 6). When the deep cells are removed from their setting by instrumentation, they often appear in loosely structured clusters wherein the structure of the individual cells may be better appreciated. Such cells are often polygonal or

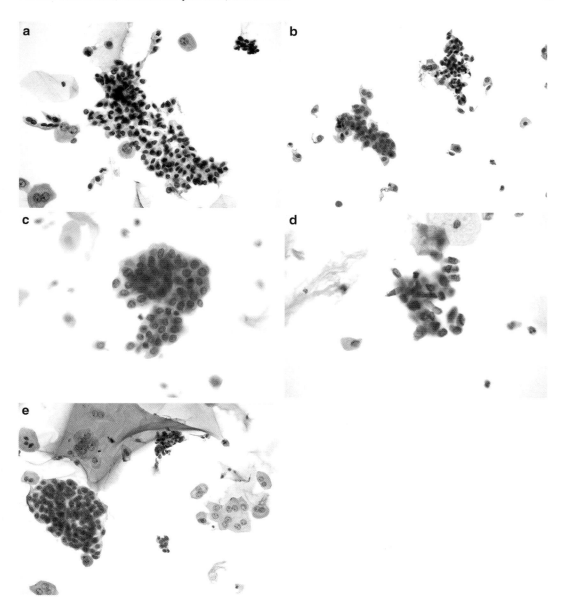

Fig. 3.8 (**a, b**) Bladder washings: Cells originating from the deeper layers of the urothelium. The deeper cells are polygonal. Their size can be compared with that of the umbrella cells in the same field in (**a**) (TP ×60); (**c, d**) Clusters of small urothelial cells from deeper layers as seen in SurePath. In (**c**) the large cluster is approximately spherical or "papillary". However, the N:C ratio is low and nuclei are perfectly round. Such cells *do not* represent a pathologic process (SP ×60); (**d**) Columnar urothelial cells in bladder washings (SP ×60); (**e**) "papillary-like" cluster of small urothelial cells from deeper layers in bladder washings (TP ×40)

elongated, sometimes columnar in shape, with dense basophilic cytoplasm and a single small nucleus. The cytoplasm may show extensions, often forming contacts among cells. The cytoplasmic extensions are the result of the tough desmosomal junctions that exercise a pull on the cytoplasm. This feature may not be apparent in liquid-based preparations (LBP).

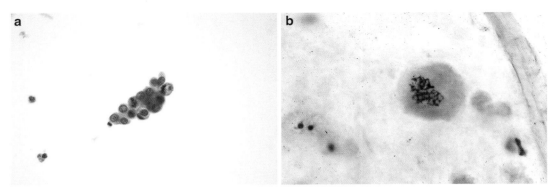

Fig. 3.9 (**a**) Mitosis in a benign urothelial cell (*center*), 3 days after transurethral resection of the prostate (TURP). There was no evidence of bladder disease (TP ×60); (**b**) Umbrella cell with finely condensed chromatin in both nuclei. The significance of this rare finding is unknown (CS ×60)

Unusual Findings

Mitotic Activity in Normal Urothelial Cells

Urothelium is one of the slowest cycling epithelia in the body with a turnover rate of ~200 days a tritiumtymidine labeling index of ~0.01%. In urinary bladder, the urothelial cell cycle time increases from 30.6 h in fetuses to 40 weeks in adults. This remarkable durability of the urothelium is functionally desirable for constant urine–blood permeability barrier. The barrier function can be compromised with cystitis, injuries such as urinary stones, surgical procedures, and instrumentation and with various drugs. Occasionally, mitotic figures will be observed in small urothelial cells, particularly after cystoscopy or a transurethral resection of the anterior prostate (TURP). In the absence of other obvious abnormalities, the mitoses reflect a regenerating urothelium and do not indicate the presence of a tumor (Fig. 3.9a).

Chromatin Condensation in Urothelial Cell Nuclei

For reasons unknown, perhaps related to some drugs or fixatives, a peculiar condensation of chromatin, resembling mitotic prophase, sometimes may be observed in superficial umbrella cells. So far as one can tell, this very rare finding is of no diagnostic significance (Fig. 3.9b).

Other Benign Cells

Squamous Cells

Squamous cells of various sizes are a common component of the urinary sediment. They are much more common in women, although there are exceptions to this rule. The origin of these cells is in the squamous epithelium that is commonly observed in the trigone of the urinary bladder, or from the terminal portion of the urethra. Voided urine sediment may also be contaminated by squamous cells from the female genital tract. Such cells may be benign or malignant (see Chaps. 5 and 6). Among the benign squamous cells one may distinguish superficial cells, characterized by a small, pyknotic

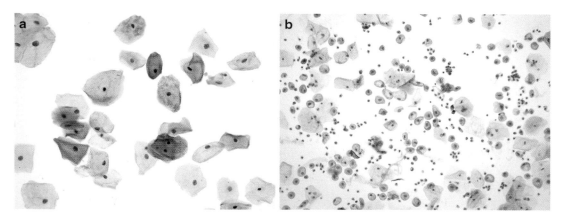

Fig. 3.10 (**a**) Squamous cells of superficial type in voided urine (TP ×40); (**b**) Glycogenated intermediate "Navicular" cells from voided urine sediment of a pregnant woman. Glycogen may not be retained in liquid-based specimens due to processing (SP ×20)

nucleus and abundant cytoplasm; intermediate cells with somewhat larger, open or vesicular nucleus; and still smaller parabasal cells. Glycogenated squamous cells may also be observed in women (Fig. 3.10a). Navicular cells are intermediate squamous cells with large cytoplasmic deposits of glycogen, staining yellow with Papanicolaou stain, and displacing the nucleus to the periphery. Glycogen may be lost on processing in LBP (Fig. 3.10b). Such cells may be observed during pregnancy, early menopause, and sometimes in women receiving hormonal therapy. They may be observed in men receiving therapy with estrogenic compounds for prostate cancer. Squamous cells may also be anucleated, fully keratinized, i.e., represented by keratinized cells of the size and shape of squamous cells, in which the nucleus has been obliterated by accumulated keratin. Under certain circumstances the presence of these "ghost" cells may be of diagnostic significance as representing leukoplakia (see Chap. 5) or squamous carcinoma of the bladder (see Chap. 6).

Intestinal Type Epithelium

Intestinal type epithelium may be the source of columnar, sometimes mucus-producing cells that are found in bladder washings and catheterized specimens but are uncommon in voided urine. The cells are usually columnar but sometimes cuboidal in shape and are characterized by clear often vacuolated cytoplasm and vesicular nuclei. Such cells may be derived from cystitis glandularis, which is usually a benign disorder. However, patients with extensive intestinal metaplasia, particularly, in extrophic bladder, are prone to adenocarcinoma. *There are no specific cytologic findings corresponding to Brunn's nests and cystitis cystica.*

Renal Tubular Cells

Cells derived from renal tubules may be sometimes recognized in the urinary sediment. These are small, usually poorly preserved cells with pyknotic, dark, condensed spherical nuclei and granular eosinophilic cytoplasm. The tubular cells are easier to recognize when they form small clusters or casts (Fig. 3.11a, b). The significance of the renal tubular cells in the sediment is not clear. In some patients these cells may reflect a renal disorder. In patients with transplanted kidney the renal tubular

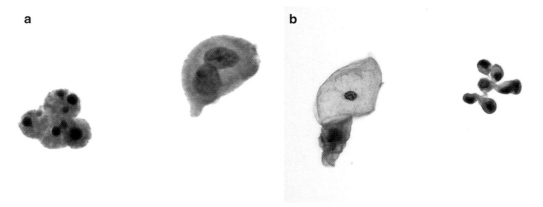

Fig. 3.11 (**a**, **b**) Renal tubular cells in voided urine: Note the small cells with peripheral pyknotic nuclei and granular cytoplasm. A multinucleated urothelial cell shown in the same field (*right*) in (**a**) gives an idea of the size of the tubular cells (TP ×60)

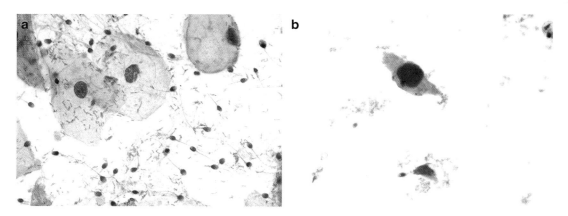

Fig. 3.12 (**a**) Spermatozoa may be seen in voided urine after prostatic massage. Rarely, seminal vesicle cells may also be present (TP ×40); (**b**) A Seminal vesicle cells with enlarged, hyperchromatic nucleus. Note the *yellow-brown* cytoplasmic lipofuscin pigment (TP ×60)

cells may indicate rejection of the allograft. Reactive renal tubular cells may show features of an atypical repair reaction (see Fig. 6.15). Such cellular changes include clusters of renal tubular cells with marked nuclear enlargement and prominent nucleoli mimicking a pathologic process.

Cells of Prostatic Origin

Occasionally cells of prostatic and seminal vesicle origin may be observed in the urinary sediment. Such cells, as a rule, accompany spermatozoa and their precursor cells in specimens obtained after ejaculation or after prostatic massage. The seminal vesicle cells can exhibit features of malignancy, including hyperchromatic nuclei, high N:C ratio and prominent nucleoli. The characteristic yellow-brown cytoplasmic lipofuscin pigment and the presence of sperm are important aids in identification. Seminal vesicle cells may also cause abnormal DNA ploidy measurements. This may be a pitfall particularly in patients being followed for high grade urothelial carcinoma. In such cases the yellowish-brown cytoplasmic pigment is essential for accurate interpretation (Fig. 3.12a, b).

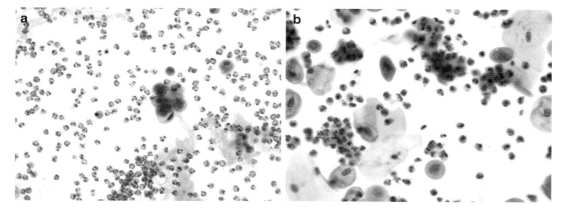

Fig. 3.13 (**a**) Voided urine with hematuria and a cluster of reactive urothelial cells (SP ×40). (**b**) Normal urine with large numbers of neutrophils. This finding may indicate either an inflammatory or necrotic neoplastic process (SP ×40)

Prostatic cells occur in small monolayered sheets or acini of cuboidal or elongated cells. Cells have distinct borders, scant amount of pale cytoplasm and round nucleus with nucleoli.

Macrophages

Macrophages or histiocytes belong to the family of cells with immune functions and are therefore most often observed in inflammatory reactions. The cells vary in sizes, may be mono- or multinucleated, and are characterized by the presence of fine cytoplasmic vacuoles.

Blood Cells

Erythrocytes

Erythrocytes are a frequent component of the urinary sediment. In the presence of clinical hematuria, red blood cells dominate the sediment and may completely obscure the presence of other cells (Fig. 3.13a). However, small numbers of erythrocytes may occur, even in the absence of clinical hematuria. Although it is customarily assumed that the presence of erythrocytes in the sediment indicates a pathological condition, this is frequently not the case, particularly if the sediment is well preserved, well stained, and carefully evaluated. In such material, up to ten erythrocytes per high-power field may be observed in the absence of documented disease.

The significance of asymptomatic microhematuria has been extensively discussed in the literature. It is usually defined as the presence of erythrocytes in the urinary sediment in the absence of gross hematuria. Approximately, 6% of new consultations at a urology clinic can be attributed to asymptomatic microhematuria. Incidence of urothelial carcinoma in patients with this problem ranges from 1 to 5%.

The issue of differentiation of microhematuria due to parenchymal renal disease such as glomerulonephritis vs. microhematuria of other origin has been extensively discussed, mainly in the European literature. Morphologic examination of either very fresh or rapidly fixed voided urine sediment may allow the separation of the two cell types. Erythrocytes of renal origin are usually characterized by a dense periphery in the form of a double ring and an "empty" center. Other manifestations of renal hematuria may be partial breakdown of erythrocytes with appearance of small, irregular, oddly shaped cells. Erythrocytes of extrarenal origin may also form a double ring but fail to show the empty center. Other extrarenal erythrocytes acquire features akin to poikilocytosis with the periphery of the erythrocytes covered with spike-like excrescences.

Leukocytes

Normal urine sediment contains very few leukocytes, usually lymphocytes, and, rarely, a few polymorphonuclear leukocytes. The presence of a large number of leukocytes may be suggestive of an important event.

Neutrophilic Polymorphonuclear Leukocytes

A few neutrophils are fairly commonly seen in voided urine in the absence of significant disease, particularly in women. Their origin is most likely in the genital tract. Larger numbers of these cells usually indicate an inflammatory process (Fig. 3.13b), discussed in Chap. 5, or a necrotic neoplastic event, discussed in Chap. 6.

Lymphocytes

As a rule, lymphocytes are uncommonly seen in urinary sediment. Large numbers of lymphocytes may be observed in the presence of tumors, chronic inflammation or in renal allograft rejection. If lymphocytes are the predominant population in the sediment, the possibility of a tuberculosis, a leukemic process, or lymphoma must be raised.

Eosinophiluria

The presence of eosinophils with their characteristic bilobate nuclei is always indicative of a pathologic process. Such cells may be observed in allergic disorders, eosinophilic cystitis, which is usually seen as a consequence of prior bladder biopsies; in the rare eosinophilic granulomas; or as a reaction to drugs (see Chap. 5).

Noncellular Components of Urinary Sediment

Crystals

Polygonal, transparent crystalline precipitations of urates are a common event in voided urine (Fig. 3.14a, b). Their presence is the result of a change in the pH of urine after collection and has no diagnostic significance. True uric acid crystals derived from urinary tract calculi are exceedingly rare. From time to time other crystals may be observed but they are very rarely of diagnostic value. The

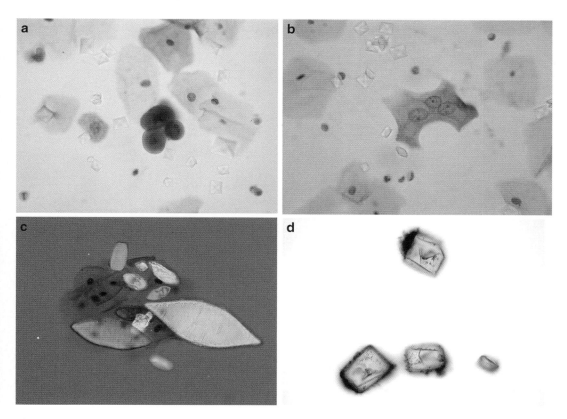

Fig. 3.14 (**a**, **b**) Voided urine with urate crystals and reactive urothelial cells (**a**, **b**, SP ×60); (**c**) Voided urine with uric acid crystals under polarizing light microscopy (TP ×40) and (**d**) calcium oxalate crystals in voided urine (TP ×60)

classic uric acid crystals are thin rhombus-shaped plates with more or less eroded tops. The other forms are the hexagonal plate, the needle, and the rosette. Uric acid crystals usually have a character-istic yellow color. The intensity of the color depends on the thickness of the crystal, thus very thin plates seem colorless, while the massive crystals have a color that tends to be brown (Fig. 3.14c). Calcium carbonate crystals usually appear as large yellow-brown or colorless spheroids with radial striations. They can also be seen as smaller crystals with round, ovoid, or dumbbell shapes. Calcium oxalate crystals are shown (Fig. 3.14d).

Contaminants

Voided urine, and sometimes specimens obtained by means of instrumentation, may contain crystals of surgical powder or cotton threads. Rarely other contaminants, such as the brown fungus of the spe-cies Alternaria, a common laboratory contaminant, may be observed. Its oval brown, septated spores are easy to recognize (Fig. 3.15a). Corpora amylacea are condensed secretions of prostatic glands that may become calcified ("prostatic stones"). They appear as acellular lamillated basophilic structures

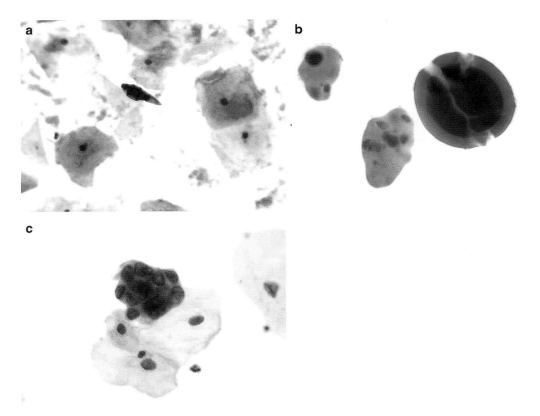

Fig. 3.15 Contaminants. (**a**) Voided urine with Alternaria that may represent contamination from water supply (TP ×40); (**b**) Voided urine with corpora amylacea. Note concentric lamellations (TP ×60); (**c**) Benign endometrial cells may be seen in voided urine in women as part of vaginal contamination and appear similar to those seen in Pap test. Note resemblance to small urothelial cells cluster in Fig. 3.8c. Correlation with menstrual history may be prudent (TP ×60)

from men after ejaculation or prostatic massage. They are of no clinical significance (Fig. 3.15b). Rarely, benign endometrial cells may present in urine cytology due to vaginal contamination. Correlation with menstrual history would be prudent (Fig. 3.15c).

Renal Casts

Depending on the methods of collection and processing of the urinary sediment, renal casts may be observed in variable numbers. The casts may be hyaline, granular, or cellular. The hyaline casts are cylinders of variable length composed of a transparent, homogenous protein precipitate. The granular casts are usually casts composed of the remnants of the granular cytoplasm of renal tubular cells that can no longer be identified. The cellular casts are composed of renal tubular cells. It is generally assumed in the medical literature that the presence of casts in the urinary sediment is an important indication of a serious disorder of the kidney. However, a small number of renal casts is commonly observed in healthy patients without any evidence of renal disease. It is likely that these casts represent a normal turnover of the renal epithelial tubular cells (Fig. 3.16a–c).

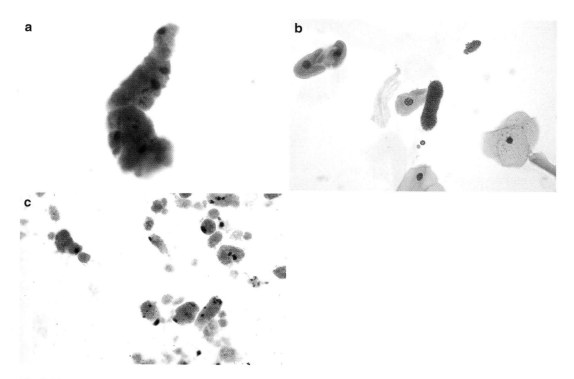

Fig. 3.16 (**a**) Renal tubular cells forming casts in voided urine. Note small cells with a small, round, pyknotic nucleus, and granular cytoplasm (TP ×60); (**b**, **c**) Granular cell cast and renal tubular cell cast, voided urine (**b**, SP ×40 and **c**, CS ×40)

Suggested Readings

1. Ali SA, Rosenthal DL, Ali TZ, Epstein JI. Atlas of Urinary Cytopathology with Histopathologic Correlation. New York, NY: Demos Medical; 2010.
2. Bardales RH. Practical Urologic Cytopathology. New York, NY: Oxford University Press; 2002.
3. Cordon-Cardo C, Bander NH, Fradet Y, et al. Immunoanatomic dissection of the human urinary tract by monoclonal antibodies. Histochem Cytochem. 1984;32:1035–40.
4. Cordon-Cardo C, Finstad CL, Bander NH, et al. Immunoanatomic distribution of cytostructural and tissue-associated antigens in the human urinary tract. Am J Pathol. 1987;126:269–84.
5. Feifer AH, Steinberg J, Tanguay S, et al. The prevalence and significance of Brunn's nests, cystitis cystica and Squamous metaplasia in normal bladders. J Urol. 1979;122:317–21.
6. Foot NC. Glandular metaplasia of the epithelium of the urinary tract. South Med. 1944;37:137–42.
7. Farsund T. Preparation of bladder mucosa for micro-flow fluorometry. Virchows Arch B Cell Pathol Incl Mol Pathol. 1974;16:35–42.
8. Golin AL, Howard RS. Asymptomatic microscopic hematuria. J Urol. 1980;124:389–91.
9. Gutmann EJ. Seminal vesicle cell in a spontaneously voided urine. Diagn Cytopathol. 2006;34:824–5.
10. Hicks RM. The function of the Golgi complex in transitional epithelium. Synthesis of the thick cell membrane. J Cell Biol. 1966;30:623–43.
11. Ito N, Hirose M, Shirai T, et al. Lesions of the urinary bladder epithelium in 125 autopsy cases. Acta Pathol Jpn. 1981;31:545–57.
12. Jacob J, Ludgate CM, Forde J, et al. Recent observations on the ultrastructure of human urothelium. 1. Normal bladder of elderly subjects. Cell Tiss Res. 1978;543:543–60.
13. Kassouf W. Utility of urine cytology in the workup of asymptomatic microscopic hematuria in low-risk patients. Urology. 2010;75:1278–82.
14. Kittredge WE, Brannan W. Cystitis glandularis. J Urol. 1959;81:419–30.

15. Kiyomoto H, Haba R. Can cytological features differentiate reactive renal tubular cells from low-grade urothelial carcinoma cells? Cytopathology. 2010;21:326–33.
16. Koss LG. The asymmetric unit membranes of the epithelium of the urinary bladder of the rat. An electron microscopic study of a mechanism of epithelial maturation and function. Lab Invest. 1969;21:154–68.
17. Koss LG. Some ultrastructural aspects of experimental and human carcinoma of the bladder. Cancer Res. 1977;37:2824–35.
18. Koss LG. Tumors of the urinary bladder. Fascicle 11, 2nd Series, Atlas of tumor pathology. Washington, DC: Armed Forces Institute of Pathology, 1975, Supplement 1985
19. Koss LG, Melamed MR. The lower urinary tract in the absence of cancer. In: Koss LG, Melamed MR, editors. Koss's diagnostic cytology and its histopathologic bases. 5th ed. Philadelphia, PA: Lippincott Williams & Wilkins; 2006. p. 738–76.
20. Lin JH, Wu XR, Krebich G, et al. Precursor sequences, processing, and urothelium-specific expression of a major 15-KD protein subunit of asymmetric unit membrane. J Biol Chem. 1994;269:1775–84.
21. Madeb R, Golijanin D, Knopf J, et al. Long-term outcome of patients with a negative work-up for asymptomatic microhematuria. Urology. 2010;75:20–5.
22. Messing EM, Young TB, Hunt VB, et al. The significance of asymptomatic microhematuria in men 50 or more years old: findings of a home screening study using urinary dipsticks. J Urol. 1987;137:919–22.
23. Mohammad KS, Bdesha AS, Snell ME, et al. Phase contrast microscopic examination of urinary erythrocytes to localize source of bleeding: an overlooked technique? J Clin Pathol. 1993;46:642–5.
24. Newman J, Hicks RM. Surface ultrastructure of the epithelial lining the normal human lower urinary tract. Br J Exp Pathol. 1981;62:232–51.
25. Pantanowitz L, Otis CN. Cystitis glandularis. Diagn Cytopathol. 2008;36:181–2.
26. Petry G, Amon H. Light and electron microscopic studies on the structure and dynamics of transitional epithelium. Z Zellforsch Mikrosk Anat. 1966;69:587–612.
27. Rathert P, Roth SE. Urinzytologie. Praxis und Atlas. 2nd ed. Berlin: Springer; 1991.
28. Rosenthal DL, Raab SS. Normal morphology & diagnostic categories. In: Cytologic detection of urothelial lesions. Essentials of Cytopathology Series. New York, NY: Springer; 2005. p. 5–20
29. Shokri-Tabibzadeh S, Herz F, Koss LG. Fine structure of cultured epithelial cells derived from voided urine of normal adults. Virchows Arch B Cell Pathol Incl Mol Pathol. 1982;39:41–8.
30. Streitz JM. Squamous epithelium in the female trigone. J Urol. 1963;90:62–6.
31. Wu XR, Manabe M, Yu J, et al. Large scale purification and immunolocalization of bovine uroplakins I, II and III. J Biol Chem. 1990;265:19170–9.
32. Wu XR, Sun TT. Molecular cloning of a 47-KD tissue-specific and differentiation dependent urothelial cell surface glycoprotein. J Cell Sci. 1993;106:31–43.
33. Yu J, Manabe M, Wu XR, et al. Uroplakin I: A 27-kD protein associated with the asymmetric unit membrane of mammalian urothelium. J Cell Biol. 1990;111:1207–16.
34. Yu J, Manabe M, Sun TT. Identification of an 85-100-KD glycoprotein as a cell surface marker for an advanced stage of urothelial differentiation association with inter-plaque ('hinge') area. Epithelial Cell Biol. 1992;1:4–12.

Chapter 4
The Cytologic Makeup of the Urinary Sediment According to the Collection Technique

Keywords Collection techniques • Makeup of voided urine • Cell clusters in voided urine • Pseudoclusters • Cell preservation in voided urine • Squamous cells • Superficial umbrella cells • Urothelial cells from deeper layers • Instrumentation • Intestinal metaplasia • Ancillary tests • Catheterized urine • Flexible cystoscopy • Bladder washings • Cytologic makeup of retrograde catheterization urine • Cytologic makeup of brushings • Cytologic makeup of ileal conduit urine • Advantages and disadvantages of various collection methods

Introduction

The collection techniques used to obtain urinary specimens include voided and catheterized urine, bladder, ureteric and renal pelvic washings and brushings, retrograde catheterization of ureters, renal pelves, and ileal conduit (described in detail in Chap. 2). These collection techniques, particularly instrumentation, have a significant effect on the makeup of the urinary sediment. Catheterization of the bladder, retrograde catheterization of the ureter and renal pelves and brushings, virtually always, result in removal of urothelial cell clusters that may be mistaken for fragments of urothelial papillary tumors. Thus, a thorough knowledge of the cytologic features observed in the various collection techniques is very important in diagnostic interpretation. Tables 4.1 and 4.2 indicate the advantages and disadvantages and the cytologic appearance of urothelial cells in various specimen-collection methods.

Cytologic Makeup of the Sediment of Normal Voided Urine

Spontaneously voided urine from normal patients contains relatively few urothelial cells (Fig. 4.1a). These cells may occur singly or may desquamate in clusters. Smaller cells from the deeper layers of the epithelium are readily distinguished from the much larger umbrella cells. In voided urine, the nuclei of the small urothelial cells have a well-preserved nuclear membrane, are spherical in configuration, stain with variable intensity, and may contain visible nucleoli (Fig. 4.1b–d). The cytoplasm is scanty, often frayed at the border, and faintly basophilic. Multinucleated umbrella cells are rare in spontaneously voided urine, except after diagnostic and therapeutic procedures. Intermediate-size umbrella cells and cell clusters may be observed (Fig. 4.2a, b).

Clusters of urothelial cells may be observed in 20% of voided urine in the absence of disease. It should be noted that liquid-based processing techniques may artificially cause both clustering of cells (pseudoclusters) and disruption of large true fragments. Millipore filter processing better preserves

L.G. Koss and R.S. Hoda, *Koss's Cytology of the Urinary Tract with Histopathologic Correlations*, DOI 10.1007/978-1-4614-2056-9_4, © Leopold G. Koss 2012

Table 4.1 Principle advantages and disadvantages of various cytologic methods of investigation of lower urinary tract

Method	Advantages	Disadvantages
Voided	Non-invasive, simple, inexpensive, easily repeated, efficient for diagnosing high grade tumors and follow up of patients with treated bladder cancer	Inconsistent findings, ≥3 specimens should be examined for optimal results, low cellularity, vaginal contamination, degenerative changes
Catheterized	Greater cellularity than voided urine, free of contaminants, better cell preservation	Painful, instrumentation artifact, increased risk of infection, degenerative changes
Bladder washings	High cellularity, good cellular preservation, less contamination, diagnosis of HGUC* is easier, good for DNA measurements	Invasive, increased cellularity and instrumentation artifact may lead to an erroneous diagnosis of tumor, significant amount of gel anesthetic may partially obscure cell detail, discomfort
Upper Urinary tract irrigation	High cellularity, good cellular preservation, targeted sampling	Instrumentation artifact, value of the procedure in the differential diagnosis of space-occupying lesions of the ureters or renal pelves is very low
Retrograde brushing	High cellularity, good cellular preservation, targeted sampling	Same as above and source of diagnostic errors
Ileal bladder urine	Good for monitoring of the ureters and renal pelves after cystectomy for bladder cancer, non-invasive, inexpensive, easily repeated	Presence of benign urothelial cells may lead to an erroneous diagnosis of recurrent bladder cancer, low cellularity, poor cellular preservation, obscuring inflammatory cells and intestinal cells

*High grade urothelial carcinoma

Table 4.2 Principal cytologic features of urinary sediment according to methods of collection

	Voided	Catheterized	Bladder washings	Retrograde catheterization	Brushings
Urothelial cells	Sparse, degenerated	More numerous, sometimes in clusters	Broad variety of urothelial cells, singly and in clusters	As in washings, complex clusters and umbrella cells	Numerous umbrella cells and complex clusters
Squamous cells	Common in both sexes	Rare	Rare	Absent	Absent
Renal tubular cells and casts	Common	Rare	Absent	Absent	Absent
Contaminants	Common	Rare	Absent	Absent	Absent

tissue fragments. Clusters are commonly observed after vigorous palpation of the bladder, catheterization, or inflammatory injury of the bladder.

Urothelial clusters are composed of variable numbers of cells ranging from three or four to several hundred. Small clusters are usually flat and the cells contained therein have the same characteristics as the isolated cells. Larger clusters may be three dimensional and are often rounded and spherical (papillary) or oddly shaped, sometimes suggestive of fragments of papillary tumors. In larger clusters, the makeup of the individual cells may be difficult to determine. Nonetheless the nuclei in such clusters are usually of monotonous size and show no hyperchromasia. The periphery of such clusters should be carefully examined under high magnification of microscope. On close inspection, the edge of the clusters is sharply demarcated with a smooth "cytoplasmic collar," and the normal component cells of the urothelium may be readily evident (Fig. 4.3a–c).

The presence of clusters should not be interpreted as indicating the presence of a pathological process in the bladder, particularly not the presence of a papillary tumor. This issue will be discussed again in reference to lithiasis in Chap. 5 and in reference to papillary tumors in Chap. 6.

Voided urine may contain a substantial number of squamous cells that often outnumber urothelial cells, particularly in women. Occasional macrophages, erythrocytes, and rare leukocytes complete the

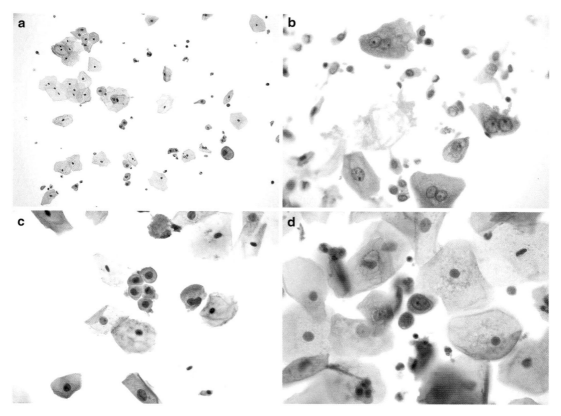

Fig. 4.1 (**a**) Voided urine. The sediment contains small urothelial cells with pale nuclei, squamous cells, and leukocytes (TP ×20); (**b**) Voided urine with single and binucleated umbrella cells (SP ×40); (**c**) Voided urine. The sediment contains intermediate-size urothelial cells (TP ×40); (**d**) Voided urine sediment with small urothelial cells from deeper layers. *Background* shows squamous cells representing vaginal contamination (SP ×40)

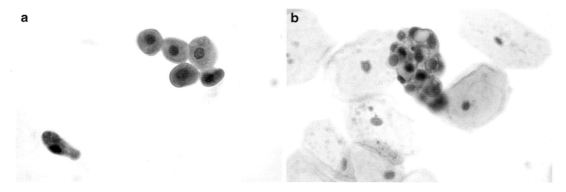

Fig. 4.2 (**a**) Voided urine. The sediment contains intermediate-size urothelial cells with pale nuclei and sharp cell contours (SP ×60); (**b**) Voided urine with a cluster of benign urothelial cells in a patient with bladder stones. Squamous cells represent vaginal contamination (SP ×60)

cytologic picture. The issue of microhematuria was discussed in Chap. 3. Voided urine may show significant changes in the morphology of cells with inflammatory and infectious processes, urolithiasis and other conditions, which are discussed in Chap. 5.

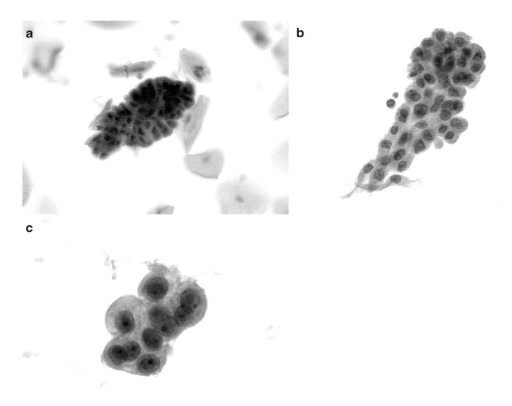

Fig. 4.3 (**a**) Clusters in voided urine may be seen without any reason (SP ×60); (**b**) and may also be seen in patients with urolithiasis or secondary to inflammation (TP ×60). Note the cytoplasmic collar surrounding the cell clusters and regular round nuclei with chromocenters in both; (**c**) Another benign cluster in voided urine showing reactive changes secondary to bladder stones. Note prominent nucleoli. However, the nuclear contour is smooth, cytoplasm is vacuolated, and N:C ratio is low

Cell Preservation in Voided Urine

Because of low pH and high osmolality, the preservation of epithelial cells in voided urine samples is usually satisfactory, particularly if the specimen is collected in a fixative (see Chap. 2). A common exception to this rule is the sediment obtained as "first morning urine," which may contain many poorly preserved cells with many eosinophilic cytoplasmic inclusions (Melamed-Wolinska bodies) that may be difficult to interpret (Fig. 4.4 and Chap. 5 for detailed description of Melamed-Wolinska bodies and Fig. 5.13). It is for this reason that the optimal urine collection should be the second morning specimen.

Cytologic Makeup of Bladder Washings

Bladder washings display a full panorama of cells of urothelial origin and offer the best opportunity to study these cells. The superficial umbrella cells are usually well represented as are cells from the deeper layers of the urothelium. Many of the cells form clusters, sometimes composed of several hundred cells. Of special significance in umbrella cells is the excellent display of the nuclear features. Specifically, the presence of multiple nuclei of variable sizes is common in the superficial cells, as is

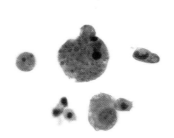

Fig. 4.4 Voided urine may show degenerative changes as shown here with poorly preserved urothelial cells with single and multiple cytoplasmic eosinophilic inclusions (TP ×60)

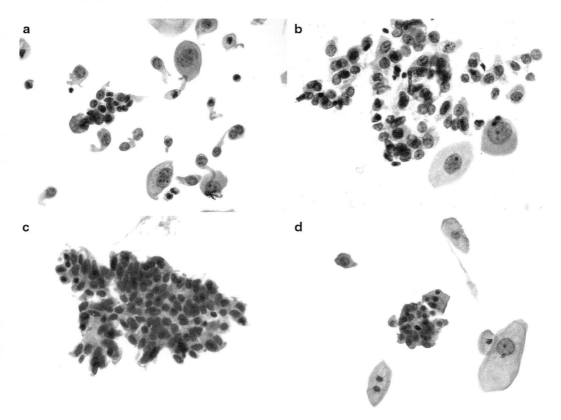

Fig. 4.5 Bladder washings in the absence of disease. (**a**) Deeper urothelial cells and mono- and binucleated umbrella cells, some with cytoplasmic elongation (TP ×40); (**b**) Deeper urothelial cells with oval nuclei and small nucleoli. Compare the size of the cells and nuclei with the superficial umbrella cells in the field (CS ×40); (**c**) A large cluster of elongated urothelial cells in the absence of disease. Note the feathered appearance of deeper urothelial cells towards the periphery (TP ×60); (**d**) Cells of columnar shape with somewhat clear cytoplasm suggestive of mucus production (intestinal metaplasia) may be observed (TP ×40)

the presence of chromocenters and, occasionally, nucleoli. All of these features are normal. The cells from the deeper layers of the urothelium are often oddly shaped because of desmosomal attachments that result in cytoplasmic extensions (Fig. 4.5a–c). Cells of columnar shape with clear cytoplasm suggestive of mucus production (intestinal metaplasia) may be observed (Fig. 4.5d).

The advantages of bladder washings are the presence of a rich population of well-preserved urothelial cells and the ability to perform ancillary tests including immunocytochemistry, flowcytometry, and molecular tests.

Cytologic Makeup of Normal Retrograde Catheterization Specimens

Makeup of retrograde catheterization is similar to bladder washings (Fig. 4.6a–c). The cell clusters may be multilayered making microscopic analysis of individual cells difficult, except at the periphery, where the features of the normal urothelial cells may be recognized. In our experience, the clusters of

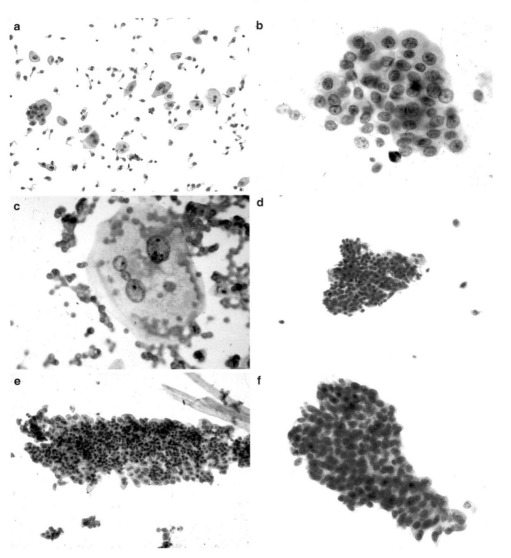

Fig. 4.6 Normal cellular components of retrograde washings or brushings in the absence of disease. (**a–c**) are renal pelvic washings: (**a**) A richly cellular specimen with many single elongated urothelial and mono- and multinucleated umbrella cells (TP ×20); (**b**) Cluster of somewhat larger urothelial cells (CS ×60); (**c**) A very large multinucleated umbrella cell (CS ×60); (**d**) Densely packed sheet of small urothelial cells (TP ×60). (**e**) Another densely packed sheet of small urothelial cells. The normal component cells are more visible at the periphery (CS ×40); (**f**) ThinPrep showing similar cytology as seen in (**e**) (TP ×60)

normal cells and the multinucleated umbrella cells, obtained by retrograde catheterization, are the most common source of diagnostic errors. Such cell clusters are often interpreted as representing a papillary tumor.

Cytologic Makeup of Smears Obtained by Brushing

As is the case with retrograde catheterization, the brush forcibly removes large sheets of urothelial cells from the surface of the ureters on its way to and from the renal pelvis, often resulting in a complete denudation of the ureteral surface (Fig. 4.6d–f). Such large clusters display the enormous variety of urothelial cells and are often mistaken for fragments of papillary tumors resulting, occasionally, in unnecessary nephrectomy and ureterectomy. It is also difficult to distinguish brushing artifact from cytologic changes of urolithiasis. On rare occasion brushing may allow localization of a high-grade tumor.

Similar changes are also seen in urinary specimens obtained after catheterization of the bladder and in specimens obtained immediately after flexible cystoscopy. These changes are transient and most disappear within 24 h after instrumentation. Cytologists should exercise caution when interpreting urine samples taken during or shortly after instrumentation, to avoid overcall (Fig. 4.7a–c).

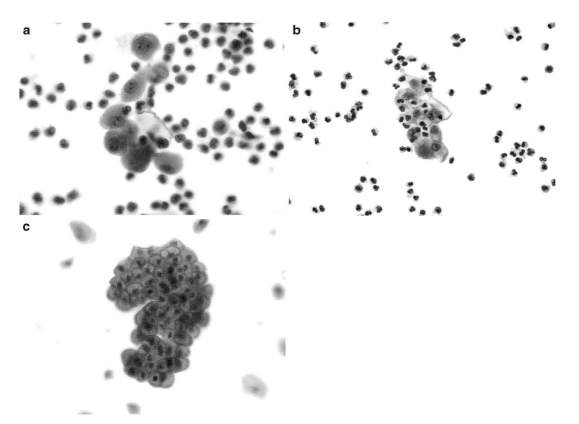

Fig. 4.7 Voided urine after catheterization. (**a**, **b**) Groups of mononucleated umbrella cells in a background of inflammation. Some umbrella cells show reactive features with prominent single and multiple nucleoli. The nuclei, however, are regular, smooth and pale. These cells could be sources of error (**a**, SP and **b**, TP ×40); (**c**) "Catheter effect" as seen in SurePath. Cytoplasm is vacuolated, nuclei remain uniform (SP ×60)

Cytologic Makeup of Ileal Bladder Urine

Ileal bladder urine is used in monitoring patients after cystectomy for bladder cancer. The ileal urine normally contains a rich population of poorly preserved intestinal epithelial cells. Sometimes these cells preserve their columnar configuration and their mucus-producing, transparent cytoplasm. Such cells usually have a small, spherical, dark nucleus located towards the periphery. More often, however, the intestinal cells are rounded, have a vacuolated or granular degenerating cytoplasm, often with nonspecific eosinophilic cytoplasmic inclusions, and fragmented or pyknotic nuclei (Fig. 4.8a–c). In such specimens, cancer cells are readily recognized (see Chap. 5). Histologically, the ileal conduit shows progressive shortening and ultimate flattening of villi and an increased number of goblet cells (Fig. 4.8d). On rare occasion, recurrence of primary urothelial carcinoma may be observed in the ileal conduit specimen.

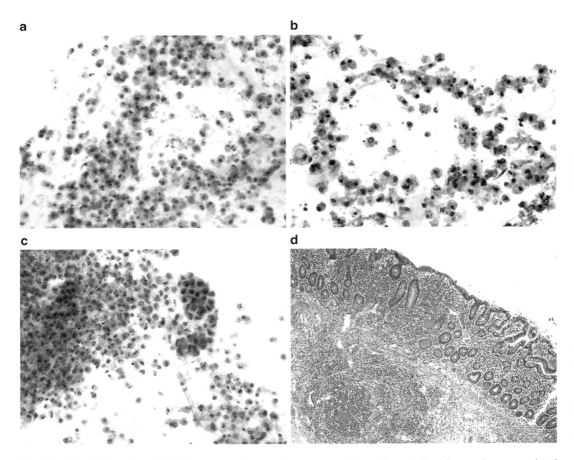

Fig. 4.8 Ileal bladder urine. (**a**, **b**) The common degenerative events are shown: the cytoplasm is granular or vacuolated and poorly preserved and often contains nonspecific eosinophilic inclusions. Occasional columnar cells may be noted (TP ×40 and ×60); (**c**) A cluster of well-preserved intestinal cells. This cluster should not be mistaken for urothelial carcinoma. Immunostains may be helpful (TP ×20); (**d**) Histology of ileal conduit with shortened and flattened villi and goblet cells (H&E ×10)

Suggested Readings

1. Ajit D, Dighe SB, Desai SB. Cytology of Ileal conduit urine in bladder cancer patients: diagnostic utility and pitfalls. Acta Cytol. 2006;50:70–3.
2. Gill GA. Methods of cell collection on membrane filters. In: Compendium of cytopreparatory techniques. 4th ed. Chicago, IL: Tutorials of cytology; 1976.
3. Harris MJ, Schwinn CP, Morrow JW, et al. Exfoliative cytology of the urinary bladder irrigation specimen. Acta Cytol. 1971;15:385–99.
4. Kannan V, Gupta D. Calculus artifact. A challenge in urinary cytology. Acta Cytol. 1999;43:794–800.
5. Koss LG, Melamed MR. The lower urinary tract in the absence of cancer. In: Koss LG, Melamed MR, editors. Koss's Diagnostic Cytology and its Histopathologic Bases. 5th ed. Philadelphia, PA: Lippincott Williams & Wilkins; 2006. p. 744–6.
6. Layfield LJ, Elshiekh TM, Fili A, et al. Review of the state of the art and recommendations of the Papanicolaou Society of Cytopathology for urinary cytology procedures and reporting. Diagn Cytopathol. 2004;30:24–30.
7. Moonen PM, Peelen P, Kiemeney LA, et al. Quantitative cytology on bladder wash versus voided urine: a comparison of results. Eur Urol. 2006;49:1044–9.
8. Maier U, Simak R, Neuhold N. The clinical value of urinary cytology: 12 years of experience with 615 patients. J Clin Pathol. 1995;48:314–7.
9. Nagai S, Murase Y, Yokoyama M, et al. Comparison of urine cytology between the ileal conduit and Indiana pouch. Acta Cytol. 2000;44:748–51.
10. Nasuti JF, Fleisher SR, Gupta PK. Significance of tissue fragments in voided urine specimens. Acta Cytol. 2001;45:147–52.
11. Talwar R, Sinha T, Karan SC, et al. Voided urinary cytology in bladder cancer: is it time to review the indications? Urology. 2007;70:267–71.

Chapter 5
Cytologic Manifestations of Benign Disorders Affecting Cells of the Lower Urinary Tract

Keywords Infections • Bacteria • Inflammation • Pyelonephritis • Cystitis • Acute cystitis • Chronic cystitis • Eosinophilic cystitis • Eosinophilic granuloma • Follicular cystitis • Hunner's ulcer • Inflammatory pseudopolyp • Papillary hyperplasia • Cystitis cystica and glandularis • Nephrogenic metaplasia • Nephrogenic adenoma • Metaplasia • Tuberculosis • Bacille Calmette-Guérin • Actinomyces • Norcardia • Fungi • Candida albicans • Polyomavirus • Blastomycosis • Aspergillosis • Viral infections • Human polyomavirus • Decoy cells • BK virus • JC virus • Electron microscopy of polyomavirus • Polymerase chain reaction • SV40 monoclonal antibody • Immunodeficiency • Human papillomavirus • Herpes simplex virus • Cytomegalovirus • Nonviral inclusions • Nonspecific cytoplasmic inclusions • Melamed-Wolinska bodies • Parasites • Trematodes • *Ovum of* Schistosoma haematobium • *Ascaris lumbricoides* • *Enterobius vermicularis* • Oxyuris • Trichomonas • Lithiasis • Crystals • Leukoplakia • Effects of drugs • Intravesically administered drugs • Systemically administered drugs • Cyclophosphamide • Busulphan • Effects of radiotherapy • Bone marrow transplant recipients • Monitoring renal transplant • Malakoplakia • Multiple myeloma

A number of benign disorders including bacterial and viral inflammatory conditions, metaplastic processes, urolithiasis, systemic drugs, and other entities may have a significant impact on the cytology of the urinary tract. Cellular changes produced by these conditions may either mimic or conceal the presence of malignant tumors. These disorders are described in this chapter, not necessarily in the order of their importance but according to their etiology.

Inflammatory Disorders

Bacterial Agents

A broad variety of bacterial agents may affect the epithelium of the urinary tract. The principal culprits are gram-negative bacteria, most commonly *Escherichia coli* (*E. coli*, 80%), *Klebsiella, Proteus,* and *Pseudomonas aeruginosa*. Bacterial infection is common in women and may be either acute or chronic. The urinary tract may be the portal of entry of gram-negative organisms, and in older adults may cause septicemia. Bacterial agents rarely cause significant abnormalities of cells in the urinary sediment.

L.G. Koss and R.S. Hoda, *Koss's Cytology of the Urinary Tract with Histopathologic Correlations*, DOI 10.1007/978-1-4614-2056-9_5, © Leopold G. Koss 2012

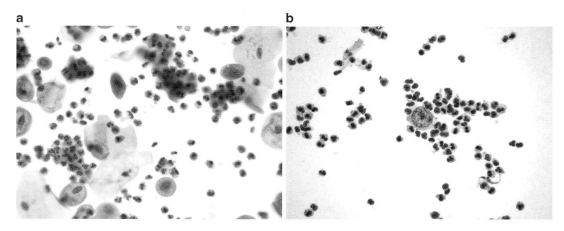

Fig. 5.1 (**a** and **b**) Voided urine sediment in acute cystitis. The background of the preparation contains numerous polymorphonuclear leukocytes and scattering of benign poorly preserved urothelial cells, some of which are binucleated and necrotic [**a**, SP ×40 and **b**, TP ×40 objective]

Pyelonephrirtis

The clinical manifestations of the inflammatory disorders affecting the kidney and the renal pelves usually are high fever and flank pain. The clinical differential diagnosis of pyelonephritis may sometimes include renal pelvic calculi or tumors, and cytologic techniques may inadvertently be used under these circumstances.

The urinary sediment may contain a large number of polymorphonuclear leukocytes, necrotic material, and renal casts composed of leukocytes and renal tubular cells.

Cystitis

Acute cystitis is usually associated with high fever and major clinical symptoms that very rarely require confirmatory tissue biopsies or cytologic examination. Disruption of the superficial mucus layer may occur. Epithelial necrosis and ulcerations may also occur. In rare cases of cystitis when voided urine is studied, the urinary sediment may contain numerous desquamated urothelial cells, necrotic material, and inflammatory cells, predominantly polymorphonuclear leukocytes (Fig. 5.1a, b). It must be stressed that marked necrosis and inflammatory cells may also occur in the presence of necrotic tumors, particularly squamous carcinoma, as discussed in Chap. 6.

Chronic cystitis appears to affect women more often than men, usually as a consequence of childbearing or obstetrical trauma. In men, chronic cystitis may be observed in outlet obstruction such as urethral stricture or prostatic enlargement.

Several histologic changes may be observed in chronic cystitis; the wall of the bladder may be infiltrated with lymphocytes and macrophages; the epithelium may show a nonspecific hyperplasia; ulcerations of the epithelium may be observed and may lead to regenerative epithelial atypia (Fig. 5.2a).

The urinary sediment in such patients is usually characterized by a background composed of inflammatory cells and macrophages. Erythrocytes are commonly seen. The urothelial cells may be abundant, although poorly preserved, occasionally forming small clusters. The cytoplasm may be granular and may contain vacuoles (Fig. 5.2b–d). The cytoplasm of such degenerated cells often shows spherical, eosinophilic inclusions that are of no diagnostic significance (see below and Fig. 4.4). Although some nuclear abnormalities may be observed in the form of slight nuclear enlargement and slight

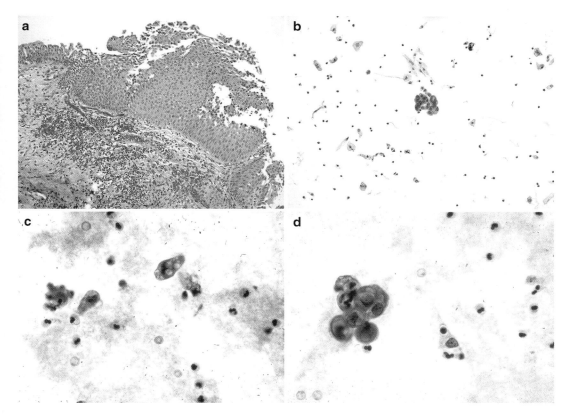

Fig. 5.2 (**a**) Biopsy with chronic cystitis (H&E ×20); (**b**) Voided urine sediment in chronic cystitis in a background of leukocytes (TP ×10); (**c**) Urothelial cells with vacuolated cytoplasm and indented small, dark nuclei in a background of lymphoid cells and leukocytes (CS ×20); (**d**) In this case of severe chronic cystitis, a small cluster of urothelial cells with vacuolated cytoplasm, small, dark nuclei with smooth nuclear membrane are seen. Cellular atypia in inflammation can rarely mimic malignancy changes (CS ×40)

hyperchromasia, the contour of the nuclei is usually regular and the chromatin texture is usually finely granular and lacks the coarse granularity characteristic of urothelial cancer cells (see Chap. 6). Very large sheets of urothelial cells may be observed in ulcerative cystitis.

Hunner's Ulcer (Interstitial Cystitis)

A form of chronic cystitis in women that is of unknown etiology, particularly unpleasant and difficult to treat is the *interstitial cystitis*, associated with chronic ulceration, known as Hunner's ulcer. We studied a number of voided urine sediments in women with Hunner's ulcer. The findings were completely nonspecific and shed no light whatever on the etiology of this mysterious disease.

Inflammatory Pseudopolyp

Chronic cystitis may result in a protrusion of bladder epithelium around a core of inflamed stroma, resulting in the formation of an inflammatory pseudopolyp. The sediment in such cases shows urothelial cells, which may occasionally show vacuolated cytoplasm. Multinucleated cells, presumably

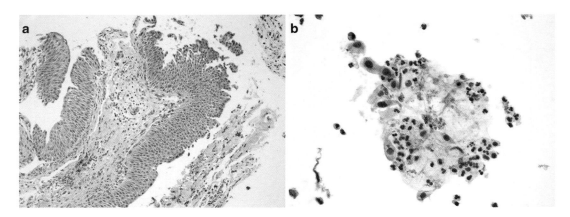

Fig. 5.3 (**a**) Bladder biopsy showing reactive papillary hyperplasia with marked eosinophilia (H&E ×20); (**b**) Voided urine from this case shows eosinophilic polymorphonuclear leukocytes with the characteristic bilobate nuclei in the background of other inflammatory cells. Eosinophils show a more basophilic cytoplasm on ThinPreps (TP ×60)

degenerated umbrella cells, may also occur. The nuclei of urothelial cells, although somewhat enlarged, show a beaded nuclear membrane and a transparent center. The background of the preparations shows numerous inflammatory cells.

Eosinophilic Cystitis (Eosinophilic Granuloma)

Chronic cystitis with eosinophils as the dominant inflammatory cells may be sometimes observed in women and children with allergic disorders. In men, the disease has been observed after previous biopsies of the bladder; or it may represent an autoimmune disorder. Very rarely, an eosinophilic granuloma may occur. The latter is a space-occupying lesion that may involve the bladder and the adjacent ureters and resemble identical lesions in more customary locations. Eosinophilic polymorphonuclear leukocytes with the characteristic bilobate nuclei and epithelioid histiocytes may be observed in the urinary sediment in such cases. In ThinPrep the cytoplasm appears basophilic (Fig. 5.3a, b).

Follicular Cystitis

In follicular cystitis the lamina propria contains lymphoid follicles with germinal centers. Follicular cystitis may be associated with inflammatory or neoplastic conditions of the bladder.

Papillary Hyperplasia

Papillary hyperplasia of urothelium can be seen overlying an inflammatory process. Urine cytology findings are nonspecific and show clusters of elongated or rounded urothelial cells with no apparent cytologic atypia (Fig. 5.4a, b).

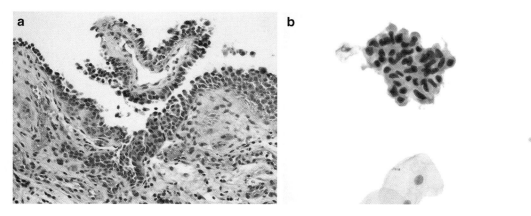

Fig. 5.4 (**a**) Biopsy showing nonspecific papillary hyperplasia (H&E ×20); (**b**) Voided urine in papillary hyperplasia showing a cluster of elongated morphologically benign urothelial cells. N:C ratio is low (TP ×60)

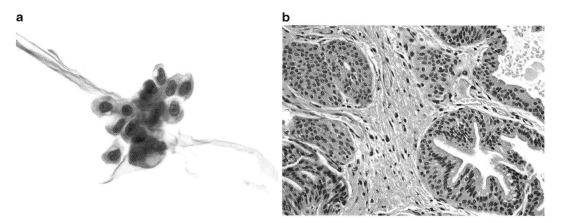

Fig. 5.5 (**a**) Voided urine in a case of cystitis glandularis. Note a group of cuboidal to columnar cells with eccentrically located nuclei and finely vacuolated cytoplasm. One goblet-like vacuole is seen. Urine findings may be nonspecific (TP ×60); (**b**) Biopsy of cystitis glandularis of typical type with columnar lining cells and no goblet cells (H&E ×40)

Cystitis Cystica and Cystitis Glandularis

Cystitis cystitica and glandularis, discussed briefly in Chap. 3, occur in 60% of normal bladders not only in the trigone but also occur in ureters and renal pelves, and the frequency increases with age. Cystitis cystica is derived from von Brunn's nests with subsequent central degeneration in these structures. In cystitis glandularis, cysts are lined by mucin-secreting glandular cells and goblet cells. It may develop as focal or diffuse glandular metaplasia of the urinary epithelium, either within the surface urothelium as a response to chronic irritation and inflammation or in the lining of von Brunn nests and cystitis cystica. Urinary cytology may not show any specific features. Occasionally, cuboidal or columnar mucin-secreting cells, with the appearance of intestinal-type goblet cells may be seen (Fig. 5.5a, b). The nuclei of these cells are regular and uniform with pale chromatin and very rarely nucleoli, which are much smaller than in adenocarcinoma. If detected in a urine cytology specimen

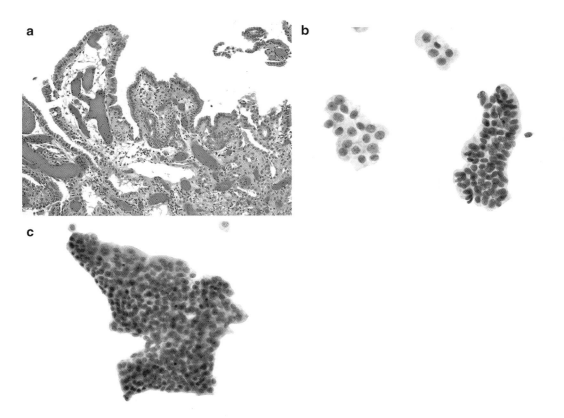

Fig. 5.6 (**a**) Biopsy of a case of nephrogenic metaplasia (adenoma) showing papillary growth pattern and small tubules in the lamina propria (H&E ×20); (**b**) Voided urine cytology in this case shows a glandular structure of columnar cells and oval nuclei. Loose aggregates of columnar to round cells are also seen (TP ×40); (**c**) Another group of columnar cells forming a glandular structure and showing uniform oval nuclei with fine chromatin and small nucleoli (TP ×60). These findings are nonspecific

cystitis glandularis should be reported. Although benign, patients with extensive intestinal metaplasia involving the urinary tract are at risk of developing subsequent bladder adenocarcinoma.

Nephrogenic Metaplasia (Adenoma)

Nephrogenic adenoma is regarded as a metaplastic process in response to chronic mucosal irritation such as chronic inflammation, prior instrumentation, calculi, intravesical Bacille Calmette-Guérin (BCG) therapy or trauma. It usually involves the bladder in adult men. It is increasingly being reported in patients with an altered immune status, such as renal transplant patients.

Cystoscopically, it appears as a small papillary or polypoid growth in an inflamed bladder. Histologically, nephrogenic metaplasia consists of papillary or polypoid structures lined by a single layer of cuboidal cells. The lamina propria shows tubules lined by cuboidal to low columnar hob-nail cells with clear cytoplasm or with signet-ring cell morphology (Fig. 5.6a). Cytologically, clusters of columnar cells with oval nuclei form glandular structures. Loose groups of cuboidal to round cells may also be seen. The nuclei are uniform with a fine chromatin pattern and small nucleoli. These cells are usually interpreted as atypical (Fig. 5.6b, c).

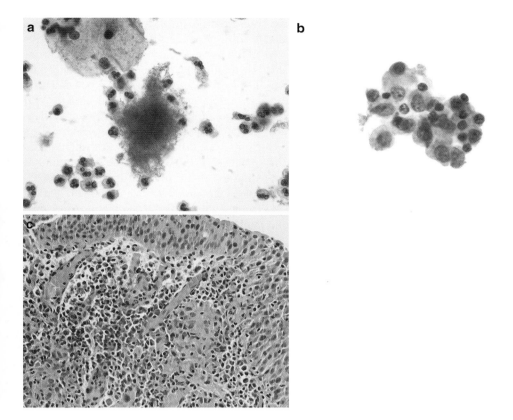

Fig. 5.7 (**a**) Actinomyces organisms are seen form tightly bound balls of slender filaments with peripheral clubbing (TP ×60); (**b**) A lymphohistiocytic aggregate representing a granuloma in a patient S/P treated with Bacille Calmette-Guérin (BCG) (TP ×60); (**c**) Biopsy showing granulomatous cystitis (H&E ×40)

Actinomyces and Norcardia

Although we have not observed either one of these organisms in urine cytology, the presence of actinomyces may be considered in women wearing intrauterine contraceptive devices (IUDs). In cervicovaginal material, *actinomyces* organisms form tightly bound balls of slender filaments with bulbous terminal swelling or peripheral clubbing (Fig. 5.7a). Norcardia may resemble actinomyces. However, norcardia are generally acid-fast positive.

Tuberculosis

Until recently, granulomatous inflammation of the lower urinary tract secondary to infection with *Mycobacterium tuberculosis* was exceedingly rare in the industrialized countries. Two recent events have changed this situation. The spread of the acquired immunodeficiency syndrome (AIDS) has contributed significantly to revival of tuberculosis as a public health problem. AIDS patients, with their low resistance to infection, may harbor not only the human variant of the organisms but also other hitherto exceptional variants such as *Mycobacterium avium intracellulare*. The second reason for increase in tuberculous cystitis is the use of the attenuated bovine mycobacterium known as BCG in the treatment of carcinoma in situ and related lesions. In patients with tuberculous cystitis the urinary sediment may show fragments of tubercles in the form of clusters of elongated, carrot-shaped epithelioid histiocytes, sometimes accompanied by multinucleated giant cells of Langhans' type, markedly reactive urothelial cells and inflammation (Fig. 5.7b, c). Diagnosis can be confirmed by a special stain for acid-fast bacilli (AFB stain), urine culture or cystoscopy and biopsy. AFB positivity by Ziehl-Neelsen stain in urine is variable and ranges from 25 to 42%. Differential diagnosis of granulomatous cystitis includes BCG therapy, fungal and protozoal infections, and foreign body reactions seen after instrumentation or biopsy. One important difference between spontaneous tuberculosis and treatment effect with BCG is that in spontaneous tuberculosis the background of the sediment shows extensive inflammatory exudate and, quite often, necrotic material. In BCG-treated patients the background of the smears is usually clean. Granulomatous cystitis with marked reactive cellular changes should not be misinterpreted as high grade urothelial carcinoma. Moreover, multinucleated giant cells must be differentiated from multinucleated umbrella cells.

Fungal Agents

Some fungal organisms may affect the lower urinary tract, mainly the urinary bladder, chief among them *Candida albicans*. Although candidiasis of the lower urinary tract may occasionally be observed in the absence of any known disease state, it is most commonly observed in pregnant women, diabetics, and in patients with impaired immunity. The latter group includes patients undergoing chemotherapy for cancer, bone marrow transplant recipients, and, perhaps most importantly, patients with AIDS. Candidiasis may be the first manifestation of infection with the human immunodeficiency virus. Unusual complications of candidiasis include the obstruction of ureters and septicemia.

The fungus is usually recognized in two forms: the yeast form, composed of small oval bodies, and the pseudohyphae form, characterized by oblong, often branching and nonencapsulated filaments with budding ends. Urothelial cells may show marked inflammatory atypia (Fig. 5.8a, b). Biopsies show inflammation of lamina propria and surrounding stroma. Fungal elements may be seen on hemotoxylin & eosin stain and if the organisms are not evident, a Gomori's silver stain (GMS) may be useful (Fig. 5.8c, d). The diagnosis of candidiasis requires a rapid clinical evaluation of the patient. In women it may represent vaginal contamination.

Other fungi are uncommon. North American blastomycosis of the genitourinary tract has been observed and the organism, Blastomyces dermatitidis, has been identified in the urinary sediment of the infected patients. The yeast form of the fungus appears as spherical structure, 8–15 µm in diameter, provided with a refractile thick wall. A single spherical bud, attached to the mother organism by a flat surface, is characteristic of the fungus. Although the organisms can be recognized in any ordinary laboratory stain, special stain, such as GMS that stains the capsule of the fungus jet black, is sometimes helpful in the identification.

Aspergillosis, a common opportunistic infection in debilitated or immunosuppressed patients, has rarely been observed in urinary sediment. The organism is usually recognized by its hyphae, which are long, encapsulated filaments, branching at an angle of 45°. The fruiting head of the organism may be sometimes observed. The diagnosis of *Aspergillus* needs culture confirmation to distinguish it from other fungal hyphae. A related organism, *Mucormycosis*, has never been recognized in the urinary sediment so far.

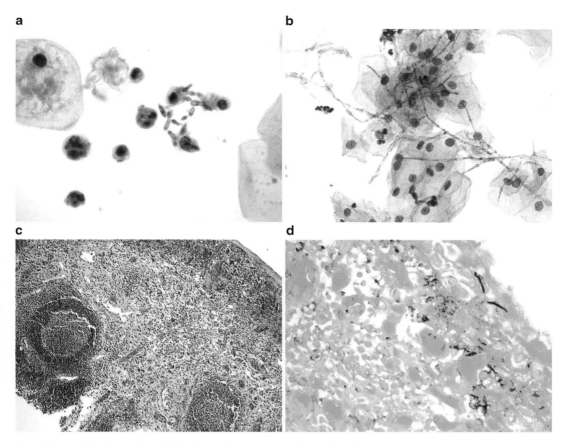

Fig. 5.8 *Candida albicans* in voided urine sediment. (**a**) Yeast form of the fungus (conidia); (**b**) Filamentous, branching form of the fungus (pseudohyphae) (**a** and **b**, TP ×60 and ×40); (**c**) Biopsy of the bladder in the case of *Candida albicans* showing mucosal ulceration and inflammatory infiltrate in lamina propria and lymphoid follicles in the stroma. No fungal organisms are visible (H&E ×10); (**d**) GMS stain show fungal hyphae (×10)

Viral Infections (Table 5.1)

There are several important viral organisms that cause significant morphologic abnormalities in urothelial cells, some of which may be confused with a malignant tumor. The dominant feature of viral infections is the formation of nuclear and cytoplasmic inclusions. Not all cytoplasmic inclusions, however, are of viral origin.

Human Polyomavirus (Decoy Cells)

Infection with this virus is widespread and serologic studies have documented that nearly all adults show evidence of a past infection. There are two forms of the virus, both named after patients from whom they were isolated. The JC virus has been isolated from a patient with multifocal leukoencephalopathy. The BK virus was isolated from the urinary tract of a patient with renal transplant. Although

Table 5.1 Viral disorders affecting the urothelium

Viral	Nuclear changes	Cytoplasmic changes
Herpes simplex	*Early stages:* "ground-glass" appearance of nuclei. Multinucleation and "molding" are common. *Late stage*: eosinophilic central nuclear inclusions.	Giant cells (multinucleated)
Cytomegalovirus	Large, usually basophilic inclusions surrounded by a large clear zone (halo) and peripheral condensation of chromatin. Small satellite inclusions.	Cell enlargement; satellite inclusions
Polyomavirus (BK type)	*Early stage*: large basophilic nuclear inclusions filling the nucleus. *Later stage*: pale inclusions *Last stage*: coarse trabeculation of chromatin.	Cell enlargement
Human Papillomavirus	Nuclear enlargement and homogeneous hyperchromasia	Perinuclear clear cytoplasmic zones (koilocytosis)

for many years it was thought that JC virus was confined to the central nervous system and BK virus was only seen in the urinary tract, it is now known that both viral types may occur in various anatomic locations. In renal transplanted recipients, BK virus may cause a polyomavirus nephropathy and sometimes even graft loss.

The BK virus plays a major role in cytology of the urinary tract because it produces cell abnormalities that may be readily confused with high grade urothelial carcinoma. The abnormalities were first recognized in the 1950s by Mr. Andrew Ricci, a cytotechnologist at the Memorial Sloan-Kettering Cancer Center, who named these cells *"decoy cells."* Subsequently the changes have been described in considerable detail.

Cells infected with BK or JC viruses are principally characterized by large homogeneous basophilic intranuclear inclusions that occupy the entire volume of the enlarged nucleus leaving only a narrow rim of nucleoplasm (Fig. 5.9a–e). The infected cells are often enlarged and usually contain only a single, spherical, regular, and hyperchromatic nucleus, but binucleated and sometimes large multinucleated umbrella cells containing inclusions in each one of the nuclei may be seen (Fig. 5.9b). With the passage of time the inclusions become pale and less basophilic and acquire a pale, homogeneous appearance (Fig. 5.9f–j). The inclusions may also dissolve, presumably because the viral particles leach out, leaving behind a peculiar network of coarse nuclear chromatin that is as diagnostic of the infection as the classical inclusions (Fig. 5.9g–l). Some elongated urothelial cells infected with BK virus are also known as comet cells (Fig. 5.9c, d, k). In many infected cells, the nonspecific eosinophilic cytoplasmic inclusions may simultaneously be observed (Fig. 5.9l). In most cases of massive infection the background of cytologic preparation contains cell debris and necrotic and inflammatory cells (Fig. 5.9d). This could pose a pitfall.

Electron microscopic studies of the infected cells disclose a crystalline network of viral particles, measuring each about 35 nm in diameter. Thus the ultrastructural appearance of the polyomavirus is very similar to that of human papillomavirus (HPV), both are DNA viruses and belong to the family of papovaviridae. There is, however, a fundamental difference between these two families of viruses: it is currently believed that HPVs of the high-risk types (16, 18, 33, 35, etc.) are carcinogenic in the human uterine cervix, anus, and head and neck organs. So far, there is no evidence that the human polyomavirus is oncogenic in humans. The cytopathic effects of the two viruses are also quite different, inasmuch as the HPV does not produce conspicuous nuclear inclusions but produces nuclear and cytoplasmic alterations koilocytosis as described by Koss and Durfee in 1956.

BK and JC polyomaviruses often remain latent within the urinary tract. Although the polyomavirus occurs in the urinary sediment mainly in immunodeficient patients, in many instances there is no

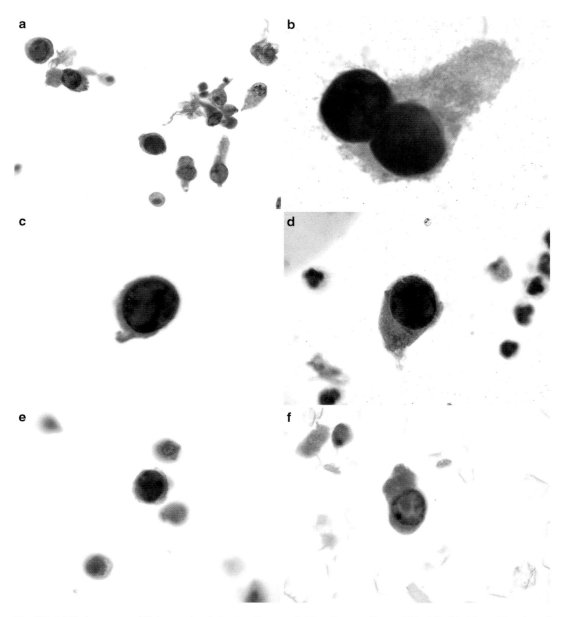

Fig. 5.9 (**a**) Various types of Polyomavirus infection (decoy cells) in urinary sediment (TP ×40); (**b**) A huge binucleated cell, presumably an umbrella cell with large, homogeneous, intranuclear, opaque basophilic inclusion. Binucleated and sometimes large multinucleated cells are not uncommon and sometimes seen in patient post-treatment for cancer (CS ×60); (**c, d**) Polyomavirus-infected cells characteristically contain a single, round, regular opaque intranuclear inclusion, which can occupy the entire volume of the enlarged nucleus. Background of the preparation contains cell debris and necrotic cells. Both cells show the classic opaque inclusion (**c** and **d**, TP ×60); (**e**) Classic Polyomavirus-infected cell (SP ×60); (**f**) Cells infected with BK virus are also known as comet cells due to a thin, eccentric rim of blue to green cytoplasm (SP ×40); (**g** and **h**) Polyomavirus-infected cells with a peculiar coarse chromatin network indicated leeching out of the virus. Also note comet-shaped cells in (**h**) (TP and SP ×60); (**i, j**) Polyomavirus-infected cells showing pale inclusion probably an intermediate stage between the basophilic inclusion and the chromatin network (TP and MF ×60 and ×40); (**k**) Voided urine specimen with massive Polyomavirus infection, depicting all stages of infection. Background contains some necrotic cells (TP ×40); (**l**) Nonspecific eosinophilic cytoplasmic inclusions may simultaneously be observed in some Polyomavirus infections (TP ×60); (**m**) Histologic section of ureter showing Polyomarvirus inclusion in superficial cells (H&E ×20); (**n**) Immunostain for polyomavirus marks the infected cells (×40)

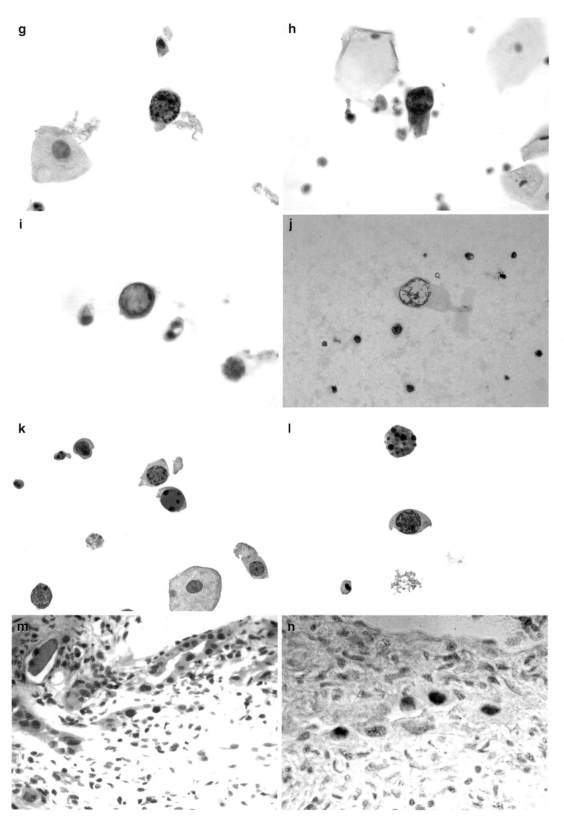

Fig. 5.9 (continued)

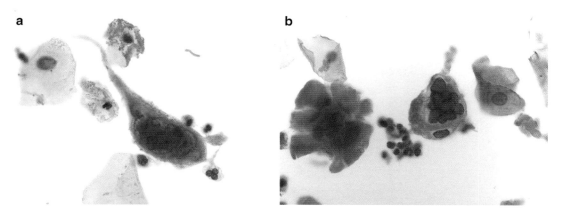

Fig. 5.10 Herpesvirus infection in urine sediment. (**a**) Ground-glass appearances of the nuclei in early stage of infection (TP ×60); (**b**) Multinucleation and molding of ground-glass nuclei in another herpetic infection (TP ×40)

evidence of immunodeficiency. The cytologic picture in such cases may be quite dramatic and has often led to the erroneous diagnosis of carcinoma.

If needed, confirmation of the diagnosis can be performed by urine polymerase chain reaction (PCR) analysis and a positive immune reaction with an anti-SV40 monoclonal antibody, prepared by Dr. Kertie Shah of the Johns Hopkins School of Public Health, Baltimore, MD (Fig. 5.9m, n). However, the morphologic manifestations of this viral infection are so characteristic that it is very rarely necessary to resort to immunochemistry for diagnosis.

Herpes Simplex Virus

Herpetic infection may occur in immunosuppressed patients, such as renal transplant recipients, in patients with tumors of the urinary bladder, in AIDS, and occasionally in the absence of any obvious disorder. Herpesvirus is an obligate cellular parasite, and florid infections with permissive replication of the virus cause abnormalities in urothelial cells that are readily recognized. Infected cells may be mono- or multinucleated. In the early stages of viral replication the nuclei of the infected cells become hazy, with a ground-glass appearance (Fig. 5.10a, b). Multinucleation is commonly observed in such cells, presumably the result of cell fusion in the presence of the virus. The multiple nuclei are often densely packed, with resulting nuclear "molding," recognized by tightly fitting contours of adjacent nuclei. In the second stage of the infection the viral particles are concentrated in the center of the nucleus, forming a bright-staining, large eosinophilic inclusion with a narrow clear zone or halo. Severe, acute inflammation may be present; consequently the infected cells in urinary sediment are often poorly preserved and the details of their nuclear structure cannot be accurately observed. In such cases specific monoclonal antibody may be used to document the presence of the virus by immuno-cytochemistry. Molecular biologic techniques that will allow the recognition of the virus by Southern blot analysis or by PCR are currently being developed.

Cells with similar nuclear characteristics may also be observed in the urinary sediment in herpesvirus type 2 infection of the female genital tract. This possibility must always be ruled out before considering the infection as primarily involving the urinary tract in women.

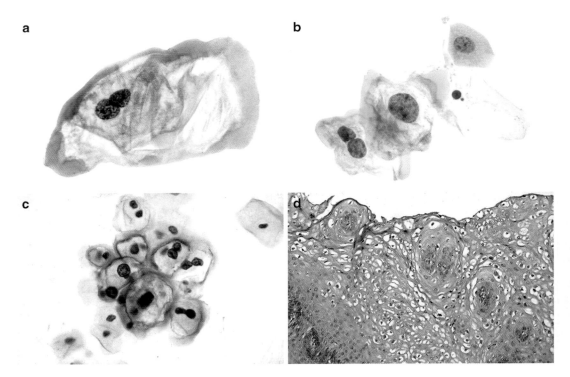

Fig. 5.11 (**a–c**) Human papillomavirus infection in urinary sediment. Note the urothelial cells with koilocytotic change and binucleation (**a**, **b**, TP ×60); (**c**) Another case of Human papillomavirus infection in urinary sediment (CS ×40); (**d**) Histologic section of condyloma of bladder (H&E ×20)

Human Papillomavirus

The current enormous scientific and clinical interest in this group of viruses is due to their relationship to cancer of the uterine cervix, anus, and oral cavity. Over 100 types of this virus have been recognized. Most of the types are associated with skin disorders and some (types 6 and 11) with venereal warts (condylomata acuminata). Condylomata acuminata may also occur within the lower urinary tract, mainly the urethra and the urinary bladder, and may cause significant cytologic abnormalities (Fig. 5.11a–d). For further discussion on HPV see section above on BK virus and also see Fig. 1.3 in Chap. 1.

Cytomegalovirus

In years past, cytomegalovirus (CMV) infection was usually seen in newborn infants, usually with fatal consequences. The time-consuming and tedious search of the urinary sediment for the tell-tale abnormalities was the standard procedure until the 1970s, when rapid virologic diagnosis became possible. With the spread of AIDS, the infection has become fairly commonplace in adults. The virus causes very characteristic cellular changes that can be readily recognized in the urinary sediment. The principal

Fig. 5.12 Cytomegalovirus-infected urinary sediment. The infected cell shows a large intranuclear inclusion, surrounded by a clear zone or halo. The nuclear chromatin is condensed at the periphery of the nucleus. A satellite inclusion is present in the cytoplasm (CS ×60)

abnormality is a large, usually basophilic but sometimes eosinophilic, nuclear inclusion surrounded by a large clear zone. There is a distinct outer belt of condensed nuclear chromatin (Fig. 5.12). One or more small satellite inclusions may be observed in the nucleus and in the cytoplasm. Cytomegalovirus infection in the urinary sediment may be the first evidence of AIDS; the recognition of the virus-induced changes, therefore, may be of major clinical consequence. As in herpesvirus, a number of virologic and molecular biologic techniques that have recently been introduced are very specific for the recognition of this infection.

Cellular Inclusions Not Due to Viral Agents

Nonspecific Cytoplasmic Eosinophilic Inclusions (Melamed-Wolinska Bodies)

Nonspecific cytoplasmic eosinophilic inclusions known as Melamed-Wolinska bodies are single or multiple, spherical, and opaque inclusions of various sizes that are frequently observed in degenerating benign or malignant urothelial cells. Similar inclusions are frequently observed in degenerating intestinal cells shed from ileal bladder (see Fig. 4.8). The eosinophilic inclusions contrast sharply with the pale gray cytoplasm of urothelial cells and measure about 12–15 µm in diameter. The nuclei in these degenerating cells mostly appear severely damaged, pyknotic, or karyorrhectic. However, in some instances, the nucleus may still be well preserved (Fig. 5.13). Although it was proposed by Bolande in 1959 that the inclusions in childhood are due to a viral infection, subsequent studies failed to confirm the presence of a virus. In 1961 Melamed and Wolinska described these inclusion-bearing cells in 43% of urinary sediments examined. They concluded that the diagnostic significance of the inclusions is limited and they most likely represent products of cell degeneration. In their study the inclusions were more common in voided urine specimens from older men, with no evidence of a specific association with any known disease state. Similar inclusions may be observed in degenerating cells of respiratory tract in ciliocytophthoria and occasionally in cells from other organs. Most patients with the intracytoplasmic inclusions have some form of urinary tract disease or injury.

Inclusions due to lead poisoning are acid-fast nuclear inclusions reported in urinary sediment of children with lead poisoning and in industrial workers exposed to lead (see Koss LG, Melamed MR. Koss's Diagnostic Cytology and Its Histopathologic Bases. 5th ed., 2006).

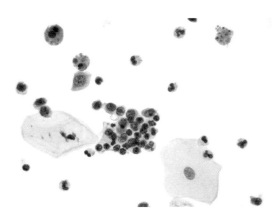

Fig. 5.13 Multiple cytoplasmic eosinophilic inclusions in urothelial cells in a voided urine specimen. The pyknotic nuclei are at the periphery of the cells. The inclusions have no diagnostic significance (TP ×40)

Parasites

Trematodes: Schistosoma haematobium

Trematodes or flukes are parasites commonly observed in tropical countries with a worldwide distribution. Most of the species require an intermediate host, usually a snail, to reproduce and infect humans. Of special interest in pathology of the urinary bladder is *S. haematobium* (Bilharzia), a parasite commonly observed in Egypt but also seen in other African countries including Southern Africa. The infection is acquired by wading in shallow waters wherein the snails reside and release the mobile form of the parasite, the cercariae, that penetrate the exposed human skin. A reaction to the infection, known as swimmer's itch is commonly observed. The cercariae penetrate the lymphatics and the venules and migrate to the veins of their predilection, mainly the veins of the pelvic plexus. The parasites mature in the venous plexus and deposit ova that are commonly observed in the bladder and the adjacent organs. The ova are excreted in urine and release a mobile form of the parasite known as the miracidium that penetrates the snail host, thus continuing the cycle. There is a known association of bladder cancer with heavy infestation with *S. haematobium*, although the mechanisms of this relationship remain completely unknown.

There are two important cytologic manifestations of the infection with *S. haematobium*: the recognition of the ova and of the malignant tumors that may be associated with it. The ova are oval structures with a thick transparent capsule, characterized by the presence of a sword-shaped protrusion located at the narrow end of the ovum, known as the terminal spine. Whether fresh or calcified (as they often are) the ova are readily recognized in the urinary sediment (Fig. 5.14a). Nonencapsulated form of the parasite, known as the miracidium, also retains the shape of the ovum and its terminal spine. Because of the movement of people across continents, associated with air travel, sporadic reports of *S. haematobium* have been reported throughout the world. The most common form of bladder cancer associated with *S. haematobium* is squamous cell carcinoma, which will be discussed with other bladder tumors in Chap. 6.

Other Parasites

Ova of other parasites may be occasionally recognized in the urinary sediment including ova of common intestinal parasites such as *Ascaris lumbricoides* and *Enterobius vermicularis* (Oxyuris). Trichomonas rarely involves the bladder. In women it is usually a vaginal contaminant and in men it

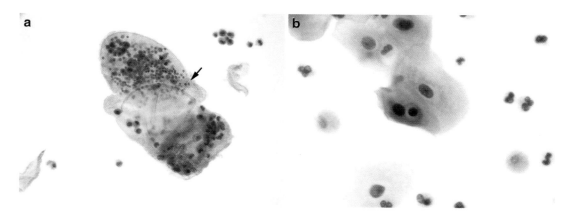

Fig. 5.14 (**a**) Voided urine from a visitor from Egypt shows an ovum of *Schistosoma haematobium*. The ovum is oval with a thick transparent capsule and shows a terminal spine (*arrow*). Multinucleated giant cells surround the ovum (TP ×60); (**b**) Two trichomonads in a voided urine specimen in a woman representing vaginal contamination (TP ×60)

may be seen in the urethra where it causes nongonococcal urethritis. Cytologically, the organisms appear similar to those seen in cervicovaginal smears (Fig. 5.14b).

Lithiasis

Pain and gross hematuria are the usual clinical symptoms associated with lithiasis. Urolithiasis is a common cause of cell clusters leading to diagnostic errors. Stones, located anywhere in the lower urinary tract, may act as abrasive instruments and dislodge epithelial fragments that sometimes may be quite large and have the "papillary" morphologic appearance that may mimic fragments of papillary tumors. Cytologically, the background of the preparation may show inflammation and blood, occasional crystals or calcifications with dispersed pseudopapillary clusters of urothelial cells. These clusters are composed of moderate-sized urothelial cells and have no connective tissue core and therefore should be considered pseudopapillary. The clusters are spherical, three-dimensional with a smooth contour and peripheral cytoplasmic rim or collar. Occasionally crystals may be seen embedded within the clusters. Nuclei may be enlarged, smooth, and round with prominent nucleoli. Degenerative nuclear changes, in the form of chromatin granularity, may occur (Fig. 5.15a–j). Patients with calculi may also have concurrent urothelial carcinoma and further investigation should be suggested after removal of calculus if cytology is of concern.

Leukoplakia

Leukoplakia of the bladder is a condition of partial or complete keratinization of the bladder epithelium, with resulting white appearance on cystoscopic inspection. Leukoplakia may be associated with lithiasis but quite often no known cause of this disorder can be identified. On microscopic examination, the urothelium in leukoplakia is provided with a thick layer of surface keratin. In the urinary sediment, anucleated keratinized cells (ghost cells) may be evident (Fig. 5.16). Leukoplakia per se is

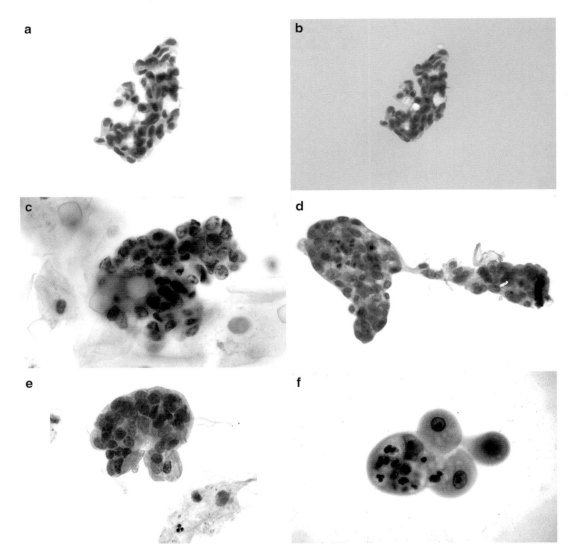

Fig. 5.15 Lithiasis in the bladder. (**a**) Three-dimensional or "papillary-like" cluster of elongated urothelial cells in voided urine sediment in a case of lithiasis. Vague clear crystals are visible; (**b**) Crystals are more evident on polarization (**a** and **b**, TP ×60); (**c, d**) Spherical papillary-like clusters of urothelial cells with reactive atypia in two cases of urolithiasis. Crystals are evident on conventional microscopy in (**c**) (**c** and **d**, TP ×60); (**e, f**): Lithiasis in the bladder. Note features of benign cell clusters, reactive changes with prominent nucleoli and a cytoplasmic collar (**e**, TP and **f**, CS ×60); (**g**) A large flat sheet of reparative urothelium is seen. Note embedded inflammation (TP ×40); (**h**) Histologic section in this case showed necrosis and numerous crystals (H&E ×40); (**i**) Lithiasis of renal pelvis seen in voided urine after retrograde brushing. Low-power view shows numerous large clusters and detached benign urothelial cells in the background of granular debris and inflammation. The overall presentation is typical of either a stone or instrumentation (CS ×20); (**j**) Biopsy of same case (H&E ×10)

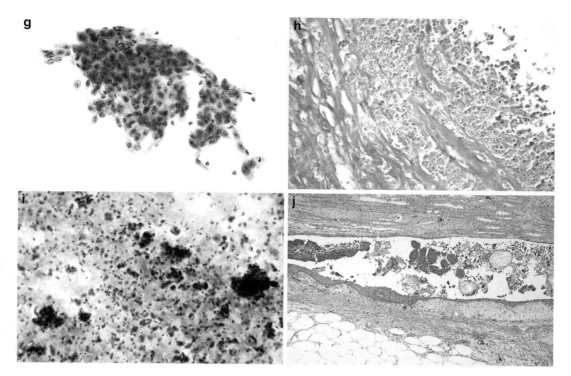

Fig. 5.15 (continued)

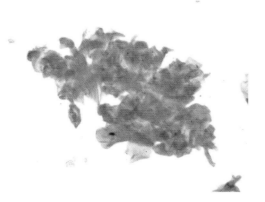

Fig. 5.16 Fully keratinized anucleated squamous cells ("ghost cells") in voided urine sediment in a case of leukoplakia of the bladder. Such cells may also occur in keratinizing squamous carcinoma. A thorough search for cells with malignant nuclei may be prudent (TP ×60)

benign but it may give rise to squamous carcinoma. The presence of anucleated squamous cells in a male patient calls for further investigation of the bladder. In women such cells may be derived from the genital tract and this source of origin must first be investigated.

Fig. 5.17 Voided urinary sediment in a patient treated with BCG for a carcinoma in situ of the bladder. Note degenerated urothelial cells and cell debris. Malignant cells are not evident (TP ×40). Also see Fig. 5.7a, b

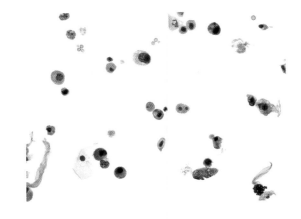

Effect of Drugs

A number of drugs administered either locally (intravesical) or systemically may have a major impact on the makeup of the urothelium and cells derived therefrom. It is of interest that, in general, drugs administered locally, for treatment of a disorder of the bladder, may have a lesser effect on the urothelium than certain alkylating agents administered systemically.

Intravesically Administered Drugs

Mitomycin and Thiotepa, are the two drugs commonly used intravesically for prevention of recurrence or for direct treatment of superficial bladder tumors, particularly, carcinoma in situ. Initially they produce sloughing and degeneration of both benign and neoplastic epithelium. If the tumor growth is controlled the subsequent effects of these drugs on normal urothelium are relatively trivial.

BCG is used with increased frequency in the treatment of superficial bladder cancers, particularly, carcinoma in situ. BCG is a vaccine derived from *Mycobacterium bovis* and initially induces a major inflammatory granulomatous response, sloughing and degeneration of urothelium. The urinary sediment may contain a large number of leukocytes and macrophages. Occasionally, the sediment contains well-formed granulomas with epithelioid histiocytes and Langhans' giant cells or dispersed lymphoid cells and macrophages (Figs. 5.7b and 5.17). Again, the use of this drug does not cause any cell changes that may be confused with cancer. Regardless of the type of the intravesical drug used, the presence of identifiable cancer cells strongly suggest that the tumor has not responded to the drug.

Systemically Administered Drugs

Alkylating agents, particularly cyclophosphamide and busulfan, may have a marked effect on the urothelium with resulting significant cell abnormalities.

Cyclophosphamide (Cytoxan, Endoxan)

In humans the drug administered in large doses causes hemorrhagic cystitis that may lead to death from exsanguination. During the regenerative events bizarre epithelial cells may appear in the urine. It is likely that a similar mechanism of epithelial necrosis followed by regeneration, accounts for

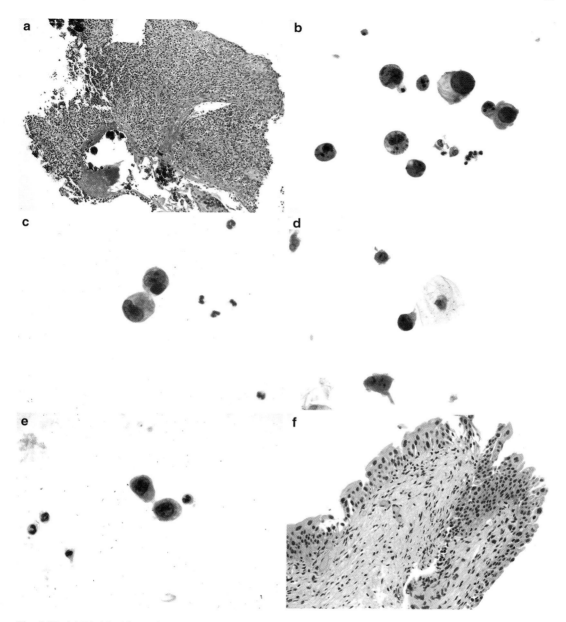

Fig. 5.18 (**a**) Bladder biopsy from a patient treated with large doses of cyclophosphamide for lymphoma developed hemorrhagic cystitis. Biopsy shows denuded mucosa, epithelial necrosis, inflammation, and calcification, a feature of cyclophosmaide-associated effect in bladder (H&E ×10); (**b–d**) Images from voided urine sediment in this patient. Note the markedly enlarged, hyperchromatic nuclei and coarse nuclear chromatin, mimicking cells of urothelial carcinoma in situ but there was no evidence of bladder disease after the acute reaction subsided (TP ×60); (**e**) Singly dispersed urothelial cells observed in a patient treated with cyclophosphamide. Note the isolated cells with nuclear enlargement, hyperchromasia and high N:C ratio (TP ×60); (**f**) Biopsy from this case shows the reactive atypia (H&E ×20)

major cytologic abnormalities in humans (Fig. 5.18a). In some cases the drug-induced changes result in oddly shaped, bizarre, abnormal urothelial cells with marked nuclear and nucleolar enlargment that mimic poorly differentiated cancer cells (Fig. 5.18b–e). Similar changes are also evident histologically as seen in Fig. 5.18a, f.

Busulfan (Myleran)

This alkylating agent is used in bone marrow transplant patients. When given in large doses over a long period of time that drug has a marked affect on the respiratory tract wherein it causes "busulfan lung". The disease consists of extensive pulmonary fibrosis and formation of bizarre giant cells in the bronchial and bronchiolar epithelium. The effect is not confined to the lungs and bizarre cells with large, hyperchromatic nuclei may occur in epithelia of all other organs, including the urothelium. In the urinary sediment, oddly shaped cells with nuclear enlargement and hyperchromasia, mimicking cancer cells, may appear. In the absence of clinical history it may be extremely difficult to identify such cells correctly.

Effects of Radiotherapy

Radiotherapy, regardless of the target organ, has similar effects on epithelial cells. Marked cell enlargement, with a proportional enlargement of the nucleus, is the landmark of the effect of irradiation. Bizarre cell shapes and vacuolization of the nucleus and the cytoplasm are other stigmata of radiotherapy (Fig. 5.19a–e). Cells with these characteristics are usually fairly easy to recognize in the urinary sediment. The effect may be observed not only in instances of direct irradiation of the target organ but also when the principal radiation beam is directed at an adjacent organ, and sometimes even when the target is anatomically distant. The cytologic findings can be correlated with histology (Fig. 5.19f). The term "abscopal radiation effect" has been applied to such events. It is of note that radiotherapy may be very effective in the eradication of invasive tumors of the bladder but that carcinoma in situ and related lesions may remain unaffected. Therefore the finding of cancer cells in the urinary sediment of patients with bladder cancer may indicate persistence of carcinoma in situ. For further discussion of these events, see Chap. 6.

Urinary Cytology in Bone Marrow Transplant Recipients

Total body irradiation and a battery of drugs, including cyclophosphamide and busulfan, are extensively used prior to bone marrow transplantation. Significant abnormalities of the urothelial cells, with combined features of radiation response and effects of cyclophosphamide and busalfan, may be observed in the urinary sediment of such patients. Biopsies of the bladder may disclose lesions that are similar to a spontaneously occurring carcinoma in situ. Because of limited survival of many such patients the clinical significance of such abnormalities is unknown.

Monitoring of Renal Transplant Patients

Urinary sediment has long been used to monitor renal transplant patients for evidence of rejection of the transplanted allograft. Presence of lymphocytes, renal tubular cells, fragments of tubules, tubular casts, and cell necrosis correlate fairly well with impending rejection. The human polyomavirus, type BK was first identified in the urinary sediment of a renal transplant recipient. The activation of this virus is a very common event in all organ transplant patients. Within the recent years other techniques have been developed to monitor renal transplant recipients. Flow cytometry of samples directly aspirated from the transplanted kidney may disclose a dominance of T-lymphocytes that accumulate during the rejection process. Direct biopsies of the transplanted kidney are also used for this purpose.

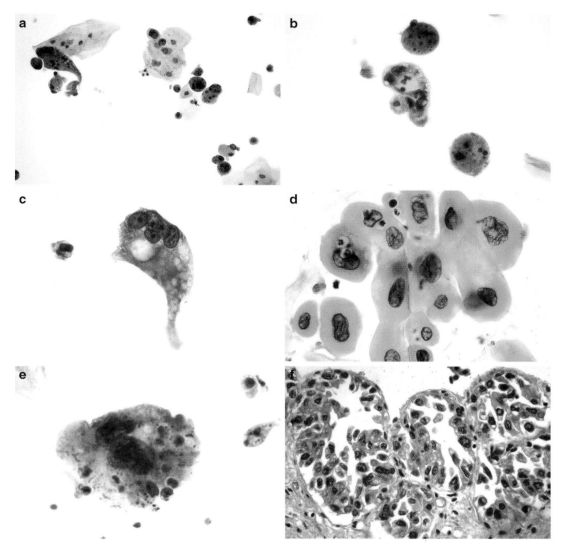

Fig. 5.19 (**a–e**) Voided urine from different cases. Radiation-associated changes display poorly preserved markedly enlarged (cytomegaly) urothelial cells with cellular enlargement, multinucleation, nuclear hyperchromasia, and cytoplasmic vacuolation (TP ×60); (**f**) Biopsy from the case shown in (**e**) showing radiation-associated changes (H&E ×40)

Rare Benign Conditions

Malakoplakia

Malakoplakia was first identified in the urinary bladder in the form of soft, yellow plaques, hence the name of the disorder (from Greek, malakos = soft). It is now known that this disorder is a chronic granulomatous disease caused by an enzymatic defect of macrophages leading to defective phagolysosomal processing of bacteria. Disease usually occurs in middle-aged or older women and may involve virtually any organ in the body including the entire genitourinary system, lungs, or brain. As a

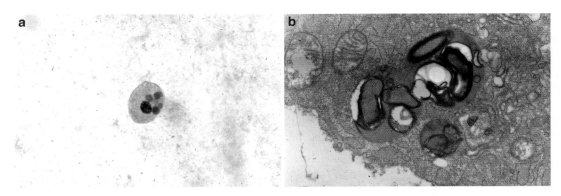

Fig. 5.20 (**a**) Urinary sediment in a case of malakoplakia of the bladder. The Michaelis-Guttmann bodies are recognized as spherical and eosinophilic structures in macrophages (CS ×60). (**b**) Electron microscopy of malakoplakia shows endocytotic vesicles engulfing *Escherichia coli* in a macrophage

consequence of an infection with these organisms there is an accumulation of macrophages in tissues, accounting for the gross appearance of the lesion. The bacteria are absorbed by lysosomes, the disposal units of the cells, wherein they remain in an undigested state. The lysosomes become very large, visible under the microscope, resulting in the so-called Michaelis-Guttmann bodies. The bodies are round, laminated and may often become calcified. The recognition of the cells characteristic of malakoplakia in urinary sediment has occurred in some instances but usually after a biopsy, releasing the macrophages into the lumen of the bladder and thence in the urinary stream. The intracytoplasmic spherical, eosinophilic, or calcified Michaelis-Guttmann bodies in the cytoplasm of large macrophages are usually readily recognized (Fig. 5.20a, b).

Benign Giant Cells in Multiple Myeloma

Globulin casts accumulating in renal tubules in some patients with multiple myeloma (malignant plasmacytoma) are characteristically surrounded by giant cells probably derived from the epithelial lining of renal tubules. In a fortuitous case such giant cells may be shed into the urinary sediment. Such cells may be readily confused with cancer cells in the absence of appropriate history.

Suggested Readings

1. Adhya AK, Dey P. Cytologic detection of tuberculosis. Acta Cytol. 2010;54:653–4.
2. Aggarwal S, Arora VK, Gupta S, et al. Koilocytosis:Correlations with high-risk HPV and its comparison on tissue sections and cytology, urothelial carcinoma. Diagn Cytopathol. 2009;37:174–7.
3. Ayra P, Khalbuss WE, Monaco SE, et al. Melamed-Wolinska bodies. E-publication. Diagn Cytopathol. 2011 May 26.
4. Bolande RP. Inclusion-bearing cells in the urine in certain viral infections. Pediatrics. 1959;24:7–12.
5. Eickenberg H-U, Amin M, Lich Jr R. Blastomycosis of the genitourinary tract. J Urol. 1975;113:650–2.
6. Gardner SD, Field AM, Coleman DV, et al. New human papovavirus (B.K.) isolated from urine after renal transplantation. Lancet. 1971;1:1253–7.
7. Goldstein ML, Whitman T, Renshaw AA. Significance of cell groups in voided urine. Acta Cytol. 1998; 42:290–4.
8. Herawi M, Parwani AV, Chan T, et al. Polyoma virus-associated cellular changes in the urine and bladder biopsy samples: a cytohistologic correlation. Am J Surg Pathol. 2006;30:345–50.

9. Jang SM, Na W, Jun YJ, et al. Primary vesicle actinomyces diagnosed by routine urine cytology. Acta Cytol. 2010;54:658–9.
10. Kannan V, Gupta D. Calculus artifact. A challenge in urinary cytology. Acta Cytol. 1999;43:794–800.
11. Koss LG, Melamed MR. The lower urinary tract in the absence of cancer. In: Koss LG, Melamed MR, editors. Koss's diagnostic cytology and its histopathologic bases. 5th ed. Philadelphia, PA: Lippincott Williams & Wilkins; 2006. p. 753–76.
12. Koss LG. Diagnostic cytology of the urinary tract. Philadelphia, PA: Lippincott-Raven; 1996.
13. Koss LG, Durfee GR. Unusual patterns of squamous epithelium of the uterine cervix: cytologic and pathologic study of koilocytotic atypia. Ann N Y Acad Sci. 1956;63:1245–61.
14. McIntire M, Scudiere JR, Gattuso P. Cystitis follicularis in bladder washings: report of two cases and review of the literature. Diagn Cytopathol. 2007;35:537–8.
15. Melamed MR, Wolinska WH. On the significance of intracytoplasmic inclusions in the urinary sediment. Am J Pathol. 1961;38:711–9.
16. Shah KV, Daniel RW, Stone KR, Elliott AY. Investigation of human urogenital tract tumors of papovavirus etiology: brief communication. J Natl Cancer Inst. 1978;60:579–82.
17. Pantanowitz L, Otis CN. Cystitis glandularis. Diagn Cytopathol. 2008;36:181–2.
18. Sulman A, Goldman H. Malacoplakia presenting as a large bladder mass. Uurology. 2002;60:163.
19. Wong-You-Cheong JJ, Woodward PJ, Manning MA, Davis CJ. From the archives of the AFIP: inflammatory and nonneoplastic bladder masses: radiologic-pathologic correlation. RadioGraphics. 2006;26:1847–68.

Chapter 6
Tumors and Related Conditions of the Bladder and Lower Urinary Tract

Keywords Urothelial hyperplasia • Reactive hyperplasia • Neoplastic hyperplasia • Inverted papilloma • Bladder tumors • Epidemiology • Risk factors • Industrial neoplasms • Aromatic amines • Carcinogens • *Schistosoma haematobium* • Cigarette smoking • Occupational hazards • Chronic irritation • Urolithiasis • Indwelling catheters • Cyclophosphamide • Paraplegic • Quadriplegic • Histologic classification of bladder tumors • Pathways of bladder tumor • DNA content of bladder tumors • Papillary tumors • Nonpapillary tumors • Low-grade papillary urothelial tumors • Papillary urothelial neoplasm of low malignant potential • Papilloma • Low-grade papillary urothelial carcinoma • Cytology of low-grade tumors • High-grade papillary urothelial carcinoma • High-grade carcinoma • Carcinoma in situ • Invasive urothelial carcinoma • Histologic patterns of invasive urothelial carcinoma • Grading of urothelial tumors • Staging of urothelial tumors • Histology of carcinoma in situ • Cytology of high-grade tumors • Histologic variants of urothelial carcinoma • Squamous cell carcinoma • Adenocarcinoma • Small cell carcinoma • Metastatic tumors • Pre-cancerous states of uterine cervix • Prostatic carcinoma • Colorectal carcinoma • Renal cell carcinoma • Distant metastasis • Malignant lymphoma • Malignant melanoma • Cytologic monitoring of bladder tumors • Reporting of cytologic findings • Atypical urothelial cells

Non-neoplastic Changes

Urothelial Hyperplasia

This is a condition in which the urothelium is thickened, composed of more than the normal seven layers of cells without nuclear abnormalities. The thickness of the urothelium may be quite variable, ranging from a slight increase to 20 layers of cells or more. The hyperplastic epithelium is well differentiated and its surface is usually formed by umbrella cells. There are two morphologically identical types of hyperplasia: *Reactive hyperplasia and neoplastic hyperplasia.* Reactive hyperplasia may occur in inflammatory or reactive processes or as a consequence of an underlying space-occupying lesion (see Chap. 5). Because the two types of hyperplasia cannot be distinguished from each other morphologically, the diagnosis depends on the environment in which this change occurs. Neoplastic hyperplasia may be the source of well-differentiated, low-grade papillary tumors (Fig. 6.1a–d). In such cases the epithelium contains branches of submucosal vessels that provide the blood supply to the stalk of the growing tumor (Fig. 6.1d). This interplay between mucosal thickening and vascular proliferation is an essential sequence of events in the genesis of papillary tumors.

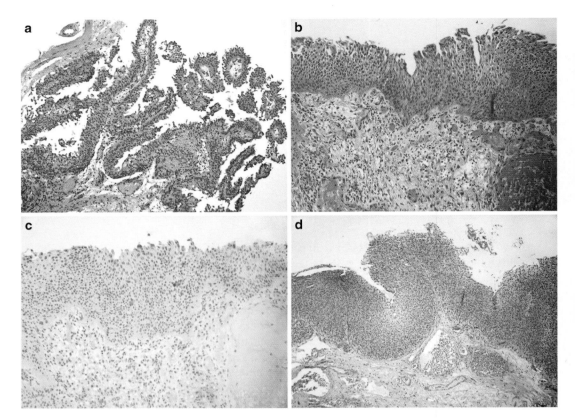

Fig. 6.1   (**a**) A typical papillary tumor with thin branches carrying capillary vessels [H&E×10 objective]; (**b**) Hyperplasia of urothelium. Note the increased number of urothelial cell layers and absence of nuclear abnormalities; (**c**) Negative CK20 in hyperplasia of urothelium; (**d**) Incipient papillary tumor. The presence of a capillary vessel within hyperplastic epithelium is the crucial event (**b–d**, H&E ×20)

Urinary sediment shows a clean background, papillary-like clusters of benign urothelial cells in an orderly arrangement. Nuclei are spherical and uniform with abundant cytoplasm. In the absence of any specific features, urothelial hyperplasia cannot be identified cytologically (Fig. 6.2a–d).

Inverted Papilloma

Inverted papillomas are rare benign urothelial neoplasms observed most commonly in the urinary bladder but also reported in the renal pelves, ureters, and urethra. The tumor can occur at any age; most patients are, however, middle-aged men. Inverted papillomas present with hematuria, urinary frequency, and occasionally obstructive symptoms. Cystoscopically, most of the bladder lesions are localized in the trigone and measure between 1 and 3 cm in diameter. Grossly, the exophytic smooth tumor appears as a polypoid nodule. Microscopic examination shows a relatively smooth surface covered by histologically and cytologically normal urothelium. The surface urothelium gives rise to endophytic cords or trabeculae of urothelial cells that grow into the subjacent lamina propria in a manner similar to Brunn's nests. Within the cords the urothelial cells show a basal layer at the periphery with features of maturation towards the center. Recurrence rate is low (1%).

Cytologically, inverted papilloma show single cells or small clusters of degenerated benign urothelial cells and cannot be recognized (Fig. 6.3a–c).

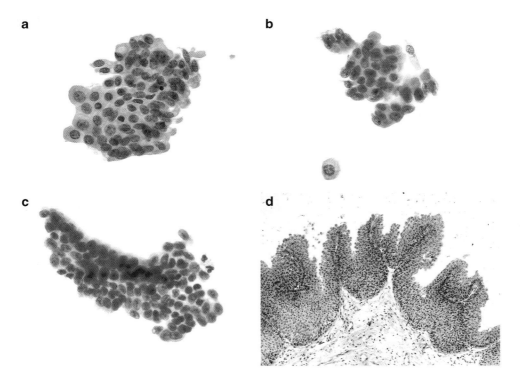

Fig. 6.2 (**a–c**) Urine sediment in a patient with histologically documented papillary hyperplasia of the bladder. Several clusters of benign urothelial cells are seen. Note elongated cells with no apparent cytologic atypia (TP ×60). (**d**) Compare the cytology with the histologic section (H&E ×20). Diagnosis of hyperplasia cannot be rendered on urine cytology

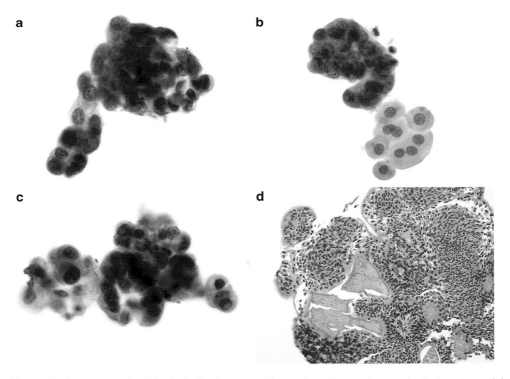

Fig. 6.3 (**a–c**) Urine sediment in a histologically documented inverted papilloma. The cells in clusters show minimal or no cytologic atypia (TP ×60); (**d**) histologic section of biopsy of inverted papilloma (H&E ×20)

Tumors

Epidemiology

In the United States, tumors of the bladder are the fourth most common cancer in men. During the second half of the twentieth century, a statistically significant increase in the rate of urothelial tumors of the bladder was observed in industrialized countries. In 2011 in the United States, approximately 70,530 people (52,760 men and 17,770 women) were diagnosed with cancer of the urinary bladder and 14,680 died of disease, according to the American Cancer Society.

Tumors of the urinary bladder are the quintessential example of industrial neoplasms, as they have been first observed and reported by Rehn in 1895 in workers employed in factories producing aniline dyes. A number of aromatic amines such as benzidine, betanaphtylamine, and paraaminodiphenyl have been shown to be carcinogenic in animals and in humans. As has been documented by Koss et al. in 1965, the development of bladder cancer is not related to dose of carcinogens. It is also of note that in most exposed workers, bladder tumors do not occur, despite massive exposure to the carcinogens. Clearly, powerful detoxification mechanisms protect most exposed people. Another important association of bladder tumors is with *Schistosoma haematobium*, a parasite commonly present in Egypt and other parts of Africa. The mechanisms accounting for this association are unknown (see Chap. 5). The dominant histologic type of tumor in infected patients is keratinizing squamous cell carcinoma that is comparatively uncommon in patients in other geographic locations (see specific section in this chapter).

Other risk factors include increasing age, particularly for white men, smoking, certain other occupations, previous cancer treatment, and chronic bladder irritation. Cigarette smoking is associated with over half of bladder cancer cases in men and one-third of cases among women. Cigarette smoke contains compounds such as 2-naphthylamine, that act in vitro both as initiators and promoters of bladder cancer. Certain other occupations including rubber and leather workers, painters, and cooks have a high rate of bladder tumors. The first three groups are likely to be exposed to carcinogenic chemical compounds, but the reason for the high rates in cooks remains unclear. Chronic irritation of the bladder due to urolithiasis, indwelling catheters, and excessive use of phenacetin or drugs such as cyclophosphamide, an alkylating agent widely used in the treatment of lymphomas and other malignant tumors, also increase risk for bladder cancer. Paraplegic and quadriplegic patients are also at risk, presumably because of inadequate voiding, and therefore exposure of the bladder to small doses of unknown carcinogenic agents contained in the urine.

Histologic Classification of Tumors of the Bladder, Renal Pelves, and Ureters

Several proposed classifications of tumors of these organs have recently been published. The tumors can be divided into the common epithelial (urothelial tumors) and uncommon tumors of other origins.

The urothelial tumors can be divided into two major groups, the papillary and the nonpapillary types. The papillary tumors are grossly raspberry-like and are classified according to the level of abnormality of the epithelium. The histologic classification of papillary tumors into low grade and high grade depends to a significant extent on the preference of the reviewer and the amount of material available for review. Multiple tissue sections are often required for diagnosis. Still the basic subdivision of urothelial tumors into papillary and nonpapillary is important because of differences in behavior and prognosis.

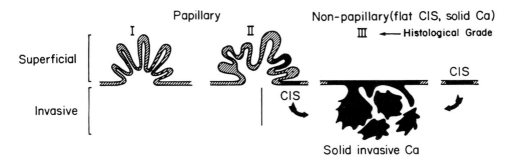

Fig. 6.4 Schematic representation of bladder tumors reflecting the morphology, grading and behavior of the two families of urothelial tumors (*Diagram by Dr. Bogdan Czerniak, Department of Pathology, MD Anderson Cancer Center, Houston, TX*)

Two Pathways of Bladder Tumors

For many years most urothelial tumors of the bladder, the ureter, and the renal pelves were thought to be malignant and were classified as "carcinomas", regardless of their morphology. Within the last half of a century, evidence has been provided that there are significant differences in behavior and prognosis among these tumors based on their morphology and clinical presentation (Fig. 6.4).

The urothelial tumors of the bladder may be classified into two fundamental, although to some extent overlapping, groups with different patterns of behavior, different prognoses and different cytologic presentation. These are:

- Papillary tumors
- Nonpapillary tumors

The papillary tumors of the urothelium have for the most part, a different natural history from nonpapillary, flat tumors. It is of particular importance to recognize that the common, well-differentiated papillary tumors (low-grade tumors) should not be classified as "carcinomas" because they do not or rarely progress to invasive cancer, particularly in young people. On the other hand nonpapillary or flat lesions (carcinoma in situ and related abnormalities) are the principal precursor lesions of invasive cancer. These concepts have now been incorporated into the histologic classification of tumors of the urothelium (Epstein et al. 1998; WHO 2004), even though they have been advocated for many years in previous editions of Koss's Diagnostic Cytology and Its Histopathologic Bases (see details in 2006, 5th edition).

Although, this simple classification of urothelial tumors is based primarily on their morphologic characteristics, it is also supported by different biologic and behavioral features that will be briefly mentioned here and are discussed in detail below and are also summarized in Chap. 7.

Of practical interest is the DNA content of tumor cells. There are significant differences in DNA content among the different categories of urothelial tumors with all, or nearly all, low grade papillary tumors having a DNA content in the normal range (diploid) and all, or nearly all, high-grade lesions, whether papillary or nonpapillary, having an abnormal DNA content (aneuploid). These differences may be used in classification of cells in the urinary sediment.

Papillary urothelial tumors, characterized by a connective tissue core, are by far the most common. Depending on the level of abnormality of the surface epithelium the papillary tumors may be of low or high grade. Occasionally the papillary tumors may invade the wall of the bladder.

Nonpapillary tumors are generally flat. The tumors may be limited to the epithelium [carcinoma in situ (CIS)] or be invasive. Mapping studies of bladder have shown that CIS is the common precursor

Table 6.1 Differences between histologic and cytologic classification based on 1998 WHO/ISUP consensus classification for urothelial tumors

Histologic terminologies	Cytology
Hyperplasia and Low-grade Tumors	
Epithelial hyperplasia	Single cells & clusters of benign urothelial cells that cannot be reliably distinguished from normal
Papilloma and inverted papilloma	
Low-grade papillary tumors	
High-grade tumors, non-invasive and invasive	
Papillary, nonpapillary, carcinoma in situ and precursor lesions	Malignant urothelial cells
Adenocarcinoma	Columnar and cuboidal cancer cells with clear cytoplasm
Squamous cell carcinoma	Squamous cancer cells

A similar table was published by Rosenthal & Raab in "Cytologic Detection of Urothelial Lesions," Springer, New York, NY; 2006. Chapter 3, p. 59

lesion of invasive cancer. There is also a relatively small group of tumors of other types such as squamous cell carcinoma, adenocarcinoma, and other cancers of epithelial and non-epithelial origin that occur in the bladder.

Table 6.1 summarizes cytologic findings in the broad variety of tumors of the lower urinary tract. It is evident from this table that cytologic recognition of low-grade tumors may be very difficult and this method is really suitable only in recognition of high-grade tumors.

Low-Grade Papillary Urothelial Tumors with no/Minimal Nuclear Atypia

The differences between a papilloma and papillary tumors of low malignant potential (PUNLMP) are subjective and may change with the number of tissue sections examined. Comparing cytologic interpretation with histology again depends on the amount of cytology material available.

Papillomas and papillary tumors of low malignant potential (PUNLMP) are composed of a fibrovascular core lined by orderly urothelium of variable thickness that shows either no deviation or only minor deviation from normal. The size of the cells increases towards the surface which is usually composed of umbrella cells (Fig. 6.5a, b). The differences between these two entities are relatively trivial: there are no significant nuclear abnormalities in papillomas, whereas in PUNLMP occasionally enlarged and hyperchromatic nuclei may occur. Mitoses are rare above the basal layer. As discussed below high-grade papillary tumors show significant cytologic abnormalities of the epithelial lining. Compare the features of papillomas and PUNLMP with those of low- and high-grade papillary urothelial carcinoma (Fig. 6.5c, d).

Because of rarity of progression to invasive cancer, the term "carcinoma" should not be used in reference to low-grade papillary urothelial tumors. Pich et al. (2001) reported that PUNLMP has a lower proliferation rate, lower expression of p53, and lower recurrence rate than low-grade papillary urothelial carcinoma. These differences are not reflected in the morphology of these lesions.

Low-Grade Papillary Urothelial Carcinoma

This category of tumors has been recognized in the histologic classification but in our judgment it cannot be reliably distinguished from PUNLPM. Low-grade papillary urothelial carcinomas very rarely progress to invasive cancer. They occur in all age groups, although they are most common in older patients. The benign nature of papillary tumors in children and young adults (up to the age of 35)

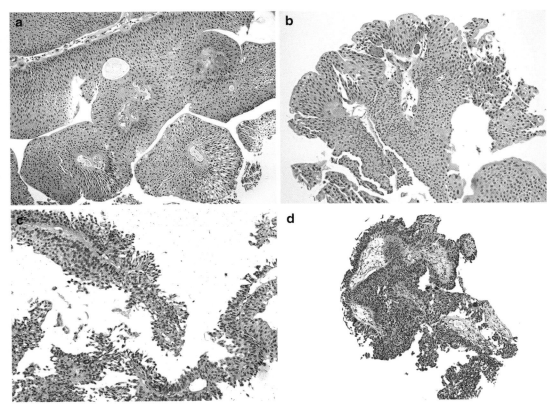

Fig. 6.5 Papillary tumors of the bladder, various grades. Two examples of tumors of the urinary bladder. (**a**) is diagnosed as papilloma and (**b**) is diagnosed as papillary urothelial tumor of low malignant potential (PUNLMP). Differences between these lesions are trivial (**a** and **b**, H&E ×10); (**c**) low-grade papillary urothelial carcinoma. Cells show moderate nuclear abnormalities (H&E ×10); (**d**) high-grade papillary urothelial carcinoma. Cells show marked nuclear abnormalities (H&E ×10)

has been documented. They protrude into the lumen of the organ, may it be the urinary bladder, renal pelvis or the ureter. The papillary tumors may be single or multiple, may have a single thin stalk or may be broad based or sessile, that is having a broader base with multiple branching stalks. Each stalk is composed of a richly vascularized core of connective tissue, supporting simple or complex epithelial folds of varying degrees of thickness and cytologic abnormality. The rich vascularity of these tumors accounts for one of the principal symptoms of this disease, namely hematuria.

Although retaining the fundamental structure of the urothelium, low-grade papillary urothelial carcinoma shows varying degrees of epithelial maturation and nuclear abnormalities that may be distributed throughout the epithelium or limited by patchy areas (Figs. 6.1a, 6.4 and 6.5c).

Cytologic Recognition of Low-Grade Tumors in Urinary Sediment

The sensitivity for detection of low-grade urothelial lesions by cytology has been generally low. In the presence of low-grade tumors (papilloma and PUNLMP), the background of the cytologic preparations is usually clean and there is rarely any evidence of inflammation or necrosis. Erythrocytes in varying numbers are usually present. Because these lesions are lined by normal or only slightly

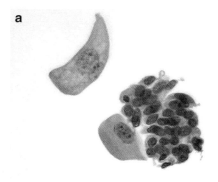
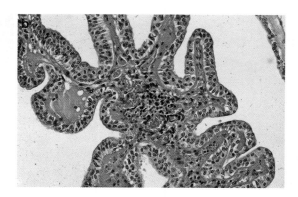

Fig. 6.6 (**a**) Normal-appearing urothelial cells in a case of bladder papilloma (TP ×60 objective). This finding is non-specific; (**b**) Compare the cytology with the histologic section (H&E ×20 objective)

abnormal, though sometimes thickened, urothelium, the cells derived therefrom cannot be identified as malignant. Urothelial cells occur singly and in clusters with an orderly arrangement. The changes in individual urothelial cells are nonspecific and the feature of slight nuclear enlargement, proposed by Murphy (2000) as a characteristic of these lesions, is not reliable because such changes may occur under a variety of benign circumstances (Figs. 6.6a, b and 6.7a–d).

Cytologic diagnosis of low-grade papillary urothelial carcinoma can also be challenging. It has been suggested that certain architectural and cytologic features may help in the recognition of these tumors. The most reliable architectural feature is the presence of papillary fragments with fibrovascular cores (Fig. 6.8a–c). However, this is a rare finding, and usually seen with large papillary tumors in which small fragments of the tumor may be seen in urine after a biopsy has been performed. Occasionally clusters of urothelial cells with irregular "ragged" edges or contour may also be observed (Fig. 6.9a–f). However, the contours can also be regular and smooth (Fig. 6.10a–c). The suggested cytologic criteria are mildly hyperchromatic, irregular nuclei, cytoplasmic homogeneity (no vacuoles) and high nucleus to cytoplasmic (N:C) ratio (Figs. 6.9a–c, e and 6.10a, b). However, these features are not reliable either and may be seen in non-neoplastic conditions, particularly, lithiasis, instrumentation and inflammation (Fig. 6.10d, e).

Cytologic features of low-grade lesions seen in the two liquid-based preparations, ThinPrep and SurePath are similar.

If the urinary sediment shows obvious cancer cells and the biopsy discloses only a low-grade papillary lesion, the cytologic finding is of great clinical importance: it strongly suggests that a high-grade malignant lesion is present in the lower urinary tract. Every effort must be made to localize and evaluate this lesion or lesions, because of their ominous prognosis.

High-Grade Urothelial Tumors

High-Grade Papillary Carcinoma

Papillary tumors of higher grades show significant cytologic abnormalities of the epithelial lining (Fig. 6.11a, b). Many of these tumors are broad-based or sessile and are lined by an epithelium that is usually composed of an increased number of layers of medium-sized cells that are arranged in a less orderly fashion with loss of epithelial maturation . Mitoses are common. In some of these tumors, the make-up of the epithelium may be identical to flat carcinomas in situ, described below.

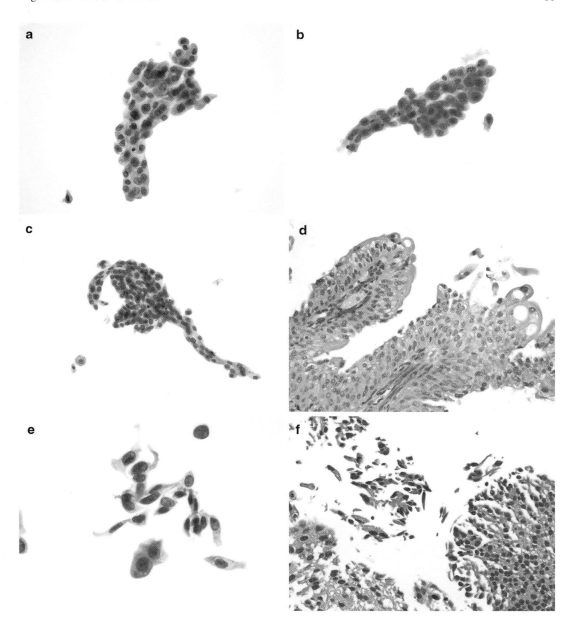

Fig. 6.7 (**a–c**) Normal-appearing urothelial cells in a case of PUNLMP (TP ×60 objective). Note the swirled arrangement of cells and mitoses; These findings, however, are non-specific; (**d**) Compare the cytology with the histologic section (H&E ×20 objective); (**e**) Another example of biopsy-proven PUNLMP showing loosely structured elongated morphologically benign urothelial cells with oval nuclei (**e**, TP ×60); (**f**) Biopsy of PUNLMP in this case (H&E ×20)

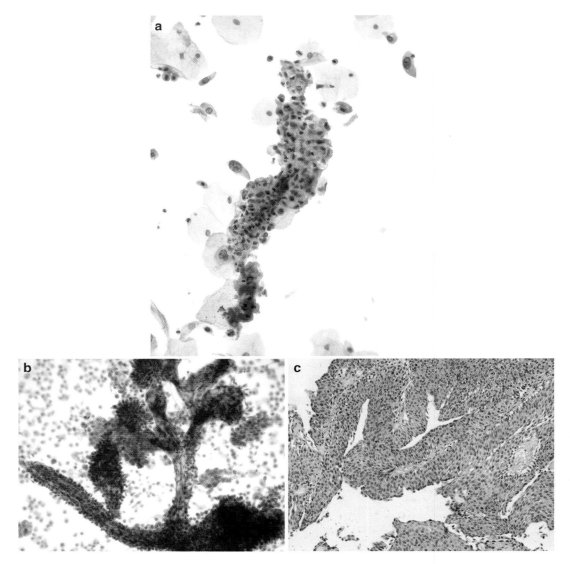

Fig. 6.8 Various aspects of cytologic presentation of low-grade papillary carcinomas of the bladder. (**a** and **b**) Low-grade papillary urothelial carcinoma in voided urine sediment and renal pelvic washings showing remarkable examples of fragments of papillary tumor with a capillary vessel. This appearance is diagnostic of papillary tumor (**a**, TP ×40 and **b**, SP ×20); (**c**) Histology of the tumor is shown (H&E ×10)

Nonpapillary Urothelial Tumors

Nonpapillary urothelial tumors occur in two forms: invasive carcinoma and its precursor lesions, namely carcinoma in situ and related abnormalities (intraurothelial neoplasia, or IUN). The emphasis in this text is on carcinoma in situ. In Koss's Diagnostic Cytology and Its Histopathologic Bases. 5th Ed., there is a detailed discussion of the precursor lesions of carcinoma in situ of various organs.

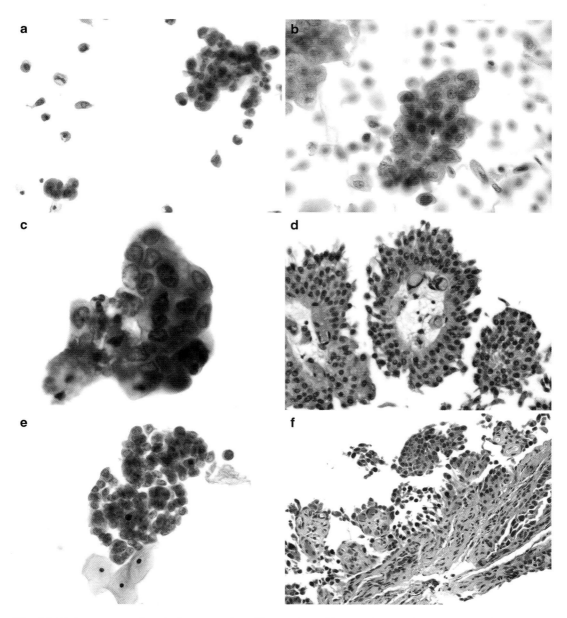

Fig. 6.9 Various aspects of cytologic presentation of low-grade papillary carcinomas of the bladder. (**a–f**) Urine sediments in patients with histologically documented low-grade urothelial carcinoma. (**a–c**) the loose structures and ragged edges of the clusters may suggest a papillary tumor, but in our judgment these findings are not specific (TP, **a** and **c**; **b**, SP ×60); (**d**) Histology of a low-grade papillary carcinoma (H&E ×40); (**e**) A complex cluster of morphologically benign urothelial cells in a spontaneously voided urine. Note the loosely structured surface of the cluster. Under appropriate clinical settings this finding may suggest a papillary tumor, however it is not specific (TP, ×60); (**f**) Histology of the low-grade tumor seen in this case (H&E ×20). In such cases a statement that "no high grade lesion identified" could be noted

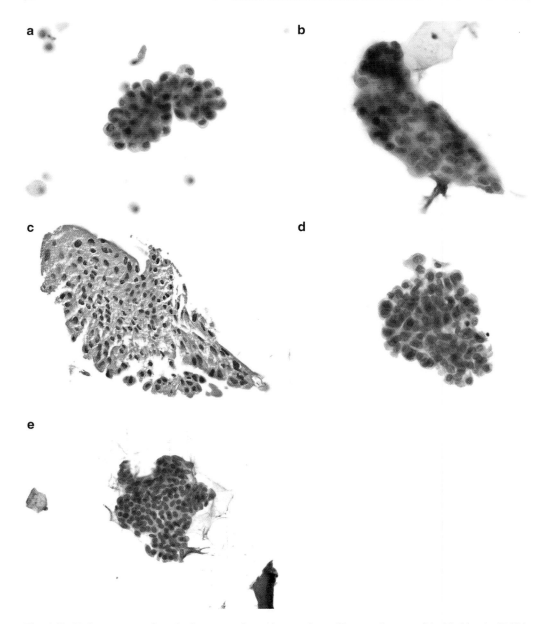

Fig. 6.10 Various aspects of cytologic presentation of low-grade papillary carcinomas of the bladder. (**a**, **b**) Urine sediment showing clusters with smooth contours and a "cytoplasmic collar" in a case of histologically documented low-grade papillary carcinoma. Both of these features are non-specific and are frequently seen in benign urothelial cell clusters (**a**, SP ×60; TP ×60); (**c**) histology of the papillary tumor from the latter case (H&E ×40); (**d**, **e**) benign urothelial clusters in catheterized urine showing the features previously described in the case of low-grade papillary carcinoma. Note the "cytoplasmic collar" in (**d**) and in (**e**) slightly ragged contour of the cluster (**d** and **e**, TP ×60)

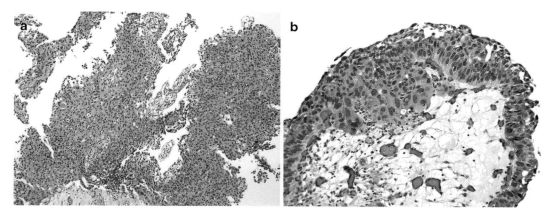

Fig. 6.11 Histologic sections from high-grade papillary urothelial carcinoma. (**a**) The tumor shows thickened epithelium with medium-sized cells arranged in a disorderly fashion and significant cytologic abnormalities (H&E ×10); (**b**) Surface epithelium of this tumor shows significant nuclear enlargement and hyperchromasia. Mitosis was also evident (H&E ×40)

Invasive Urothelial Carcinomas

Most invasive cancers of the bladder are discovered "de novo" in patients seen because of hematuria, frequency and other common nonspecific symptoms referable to a dysfunction of the bladder. It has been documented by mapping the urinary bladders, that invasive cancer is usually derived from epithelial segments showing carcinoma in situ or related lesions (Fig. 6.12).

Histologic Patterns

Tumors of the urinary bladder may have diverse histologic patterns ranging from solid or mimicking papillary tumors, to tumors composed of spindle and giant cells mimicking sarcomas, to highly anaplastic large- and small-cell cancers, the latter akin to oat cell carcinoma and other rare tumors (Fig. 6.13a, b). The most common types are derived from and retain the unique configuration of the urothelium and comprise approximately 75–90% of tumors. The remaining subtypes comprise squamous cell carcinoma (Fig. 6.13c), mixed carcinoma, adenocarcinoma and other rare cell types. These variants may be recognized in cytologic material and will be discussed below.

Tumors that arise in the part of urethra, ureter and renal pelves, lined by the urothelium, share the same subtypes with urinary bladder.

Grading

Invasive carcinomas of the bladder composed of orderly sheets of cells resembling normal urothelium are very rare (grade 1 and 2 tumors). Virtually all invasive tumors are grade 3 tumors (Fig. 6.14a, b). Immunohistochemical stains for cytokeratin 20 (CK20) and p63 may occasionally be needed to confirm invasion (Fig. 6.14c, d)

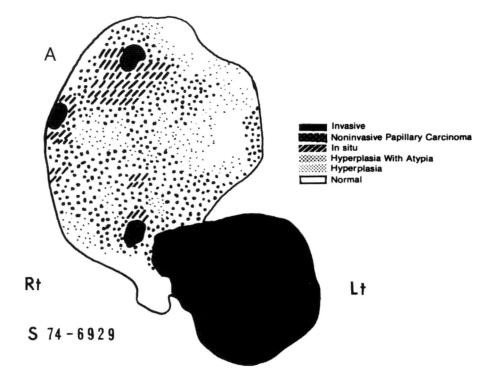

Invasive
Noninvasive Papillary Carcinoma
In situ
Hyperplasia With Atypia
Hyperplasia
Normal

Fig. 6.12 Mapping of the bladder removed surgically because of a very large papillary tumor with extension into lamina propria. Three peripheral foci of invasion are surrounded by carcinoma in situ and related lesions (modified from Koss LG, Nakanishi I and Freed SZ: Nonpapillary carcinoma in situ and atypical hyperplasia in cancerous bladders. Further studies of surgically-removed bladders by mapping. Urology 1977, 9:442

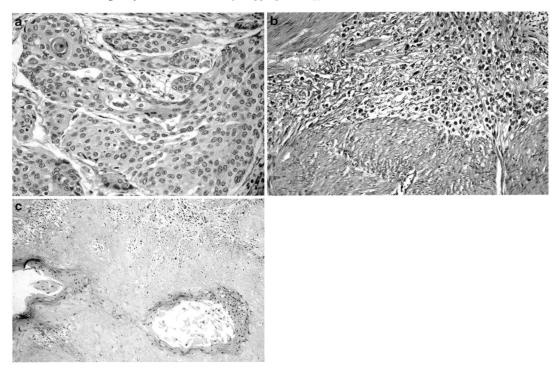

Fig. 6.13 Patterns of invasive cancer of urinary bladder (**a**, **b**) Urothelial carcinoma, high grade. The tumors are composed of sheets poorly differentiated cancer cells (H&E ×40); (**b**) Leather bottle bladder showing the presence of signet ring cancer cells in the wall of the bladder (H&E ×20); (**c**) squamous cell carcinoma with pseudosarcomatous reaction (H&E ×20)

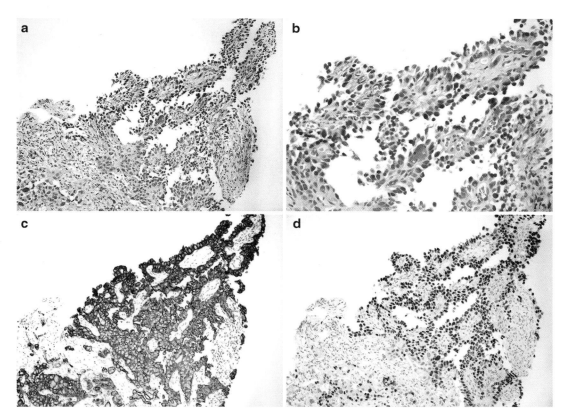

Fig. 6.14 (**a** and **b**) High-grade papillary carcinoma, suspicious for invasion (**a**, H&E ×10; **b**, H&E ×20); (**c** and **d**) Invasion was confirmed by positive CK20 and p63 immunostaining of tumor cells in the muscle (H&E ×10)

Staging

The prognosis of invasive cancer of the bladder depends mainly on the stage of the disease at discovery and the presence or absence of metastases. The diagram in Fig. 6.15 shows the principles of staging of bladder tumors. The staging is also applicable to tumors of the renal pelvis and ureters. Tumors with invasion limited to the lamina propria (Stage T_{1A}) fare better than tumors with invasion of the principal bladder muscle (muscularis propria). In the assessment of invasion, the muscularis propria should not be confused with the thin and incomplete layer of the muscle observed in some patients in the lamina propria (muscularis mucosae). In practice, tumors invading the main bladder muscle to various depths (stages T3 and T4) have a poor prognosis although there are some rare exceptions to this rule.

The left side of the diagram in Fig. 6.15 pertains to noninvasive tumors. After many years, the staging system finally recognized the major behavioral and prognostic differences between noninvasive papillary tumors, now designated as T_a, and flat carcinoma in situ, now designated as TIS.

Flat Carcinoma In Situ

Carcinoma in situ of the bladder was first described as "Bowen's disease" of bladder epithelium by Melicow and Hollowell (1952) as a microscopic abnormality of bladder epithelium, accompanying visible papillary tumors. Several years later it was demonstrated that clinically occult carcinoma in situ, identified in urinary sediment, is the principal precursor lesion of invasive cancer.

Fig. 6.15 Modified clinical staging of bladder according to the TNM system. It was recognized that there are two types of non-invasive tumors: flat carcinoma-in-situ (TIS) and papillary tumors (Ta). The two entities have unequal prognosis inasmuch as most invasive cancers (T_2 and T_3) are derived from TIS. N indicates lymph node metastases to pelvix lymph nodes (N_2) and aortic lymph nodes (N_4). The prognosis of invasive tumors depends on stage

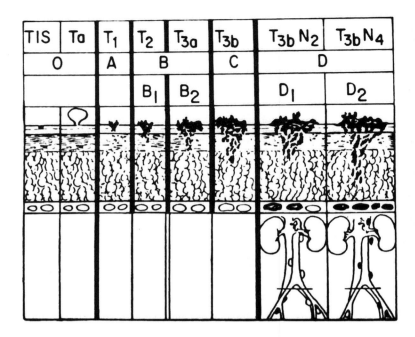

The origin of invasive carcinoma in bladders of patients with papillary tumors has also been studied by mapping of bladders removed by cystectomy for recurrent papillary tumors. It could be documented that in such cases invasive cancer develops in areas of carcinoma in situ and related lesions that may be remote from the papillary tumors (Fig. 6.16a–c). At the time of cystectomies, the existence of the occult invasive foci was not suspected. These observations have led to the adoption of multiple biopsies of the bladder epithelium as a routine procedure in the evaluation of patients with papillary tumors.

Clinical Presentation

Carcinoma in situ of the bladder may be completely asymptomatic or may cause nonspecific symptoms commonly associated with cystitis or prostatic disease. Carcinoma in situ of the urinary bladder may not be recognized as a tumor on cystoscopic examination. The most common visible alteration is redness of the epithelial surface, sometimes described as "velvety redness," caused by inflammatory changes and vascular dilatation in the underlying stroma (Fig. 6.16a). Other changes may mimic inflammation, cobblestone mucosa, interstitial cystitis, etc. However, many carcinomas in situ do not form any visible abnormalities at all. The diagnosis of the lesion depends, therefore, on either recognition of cancer cells in the urinary sediment or a fortuitous biopsy of the urothelium. The rate of progression of untreated carcinoma in situ to invasive cancer is about 60% in 5 years. The principal features of carcinoma in situ of the urinary bladder are summarized in Table 6.2.

A classical example of urothelial carcinoma in situ was the presidential candidate Mr. Hubert Humphrey who was diagnosed with this disease in 1967. He was treated with radiotherapy, known not to be effective in this disorder. Mr. Humphrey predictably developed invasive bladder cancer and died six years later of the disease.

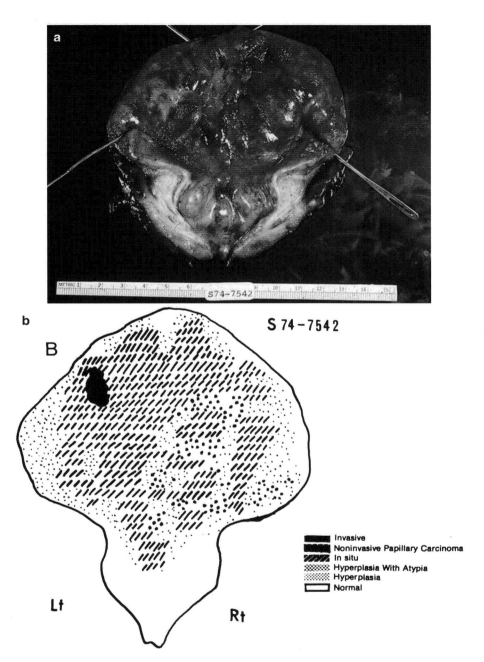

Fig. 6.16 Bladder removed by radical cystectomy for extensive carcinoma in situ. (**a**) Gross appearance of bladder with markedly red epithelium; (**b**) Mapping of the bladder showing one focus of occult invasive carcinoma; (**c**) Histologic appearance of carcinoma in situ involving nests of Brunn (H&E ×40) (modified from Koss LG, Nakanishi I and Freed SZ: Nonpapillary carcinoma in situ and atypical hyperplasia in cancerous bladders. Further studies of surgically removed bladders by mapping. Urology 1977, 9:442)

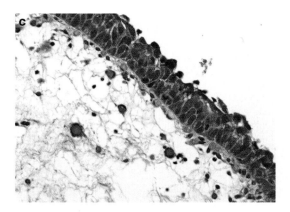

Fig. 6.16 (continued)

Table 6.2 Characteristics of nonpapillary carcinoma in situ of bladder

1. The lesion cannot be recognized cystoscopically as a tumor.
2. Cystoscopic abnormalities that may mimic inflammation, "velvety redness," "cobblestone epithelium," or "interstitial cystitis". In other cases there may be no cystoscopic abnormalities whatever.
3. In males, the lesion often extends into the prostatic ducts.
4. Because the lesion produces only non-specific symptoms or may be asymptomatic, its diagnosis is based either on cytology of voided urine or on incidental biopsies of bladder epithelium.
5. If untreated, primary carcinomas in situ will progress to invasive carcinoma in at least 60% of all patients within 5 years.

Histology

In its classical form, flat carcinoma in situ is recognized as an abnormality of the urothelium composed of cancer cells throughout its thickness. The thickness of the cancerous epithelium is variable: some carcinomas in situ are composed of only three or four layers of cells, whereas others may be composed of 15 or even more layers. The cancer cells may vary in size from large to very small corresponding to cell sizes observed in various forms of invasive urothelial carcinoma (Fig. 6.17a, b). The epithelium may sometimes show differentiation in the superficial layers and the presence of umbrella cells on the surface. Such lesions were sometimes referred to as "dysplasia or intraurothelial neoplasia (IUN)" but in our experience, the diagnosis of carcinoma in situ can be established even if the malignant cells are confined to three or four basal layers of the epithelium. We also observed a case of carcinoma in situ of the bladder composed of large cancer cells with eosinophilic cytoplasm, resembling oncocytes. Extension of carcinoma in situ into the nests of von Brunn should not be considered as evidence of invasion (Fig. 6.17b).

Because the cancerous epithelium is fragile, sometimes only the frayed remains of bottom layers may be observed in the biopsy (Fig. 6.17c). The term "denuding cystitis" or, more recently, "clinging variant of carcinoma in situ" has been proposed to describe this phenomenon.

Another form of carcinoma in situ may mimic Paget's disease of the breast and is characterized by the presence of large cancer cells with clear cytoplasm (Fig. 6.17d). It is of note that the pattern of Paget's disease is repeated in the epithelia of the vulva, vagina, and penis in metastatic urothelial carcinoma to these organs.

Carcinoma in situ may be multicentric and involve several areas of the urothelium. As documented by biopsies of workers exposed to carcinogens, these lesions were most often observed in the floor of

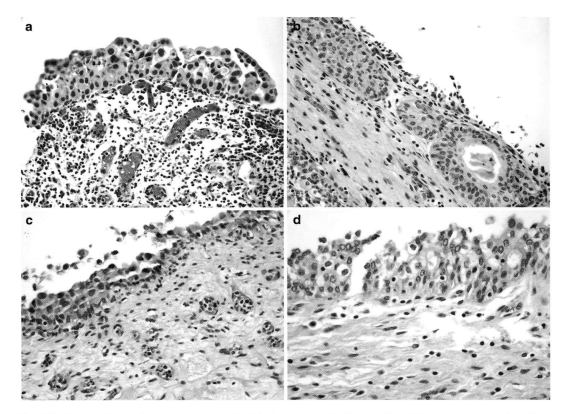

Fig. 6.17 Various forms of carcinoma in situ. (**a**) A lesion composed of large cells; (**b**) lesion composed of medium-sized cells involving von Brunn's nest; (**c**) Lesion showing small cells attached to the surface of the bladder (**a–c**, H&E ×20); (**d**) pagetoid-type of carcinoma in situ (H&E ×40)

the bladder (the trigone area), including the periureteral areas, followed by bladder neck. The posterior and lateral walls of the bladder were next in frequency of involvement. The anterior wall or the dome was rarely involved.

Carcinoma in situ may extend to the distal ureters and the urethra in both female and male patients. An extension of carcinoma in situ of the bladder into the prostatic ducts is an important complication of this disease. This has a major impact on treatment options because the tumor in the prostatic ducts is not accessible to and does not respond to immunotherapy with bacillus Calmette-Guerin (BCG).

Cytologic Recognition of High-Grade Urothelial Tumors in Urinary Sediment

All or nearly all high-grade urothelial carcinomas can be identified by cytology. Voided urine sediment is the ideal diagnostic medium for primary diagnosis of high-grade carcinoma, whether located in the bladder, the renal pelvis or the ureters. The cytology of high-grade lesions including high-grade papillary, nonpapillary invasive carcinoma and carcinoma in situ is identical or similar. The background however, may be different. In carcinoma in situ, the background rarely contains more than a few inflammatory cells or erythrocytes, and there is usually little evidence of necrosis, whereas marked

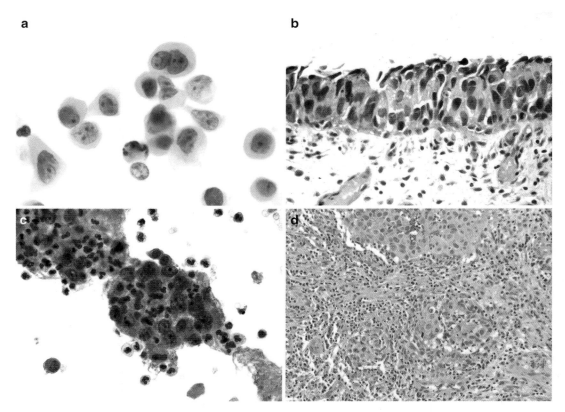

Fig. 6.18 Comparison of carcinoma in situ and invasive carcinoma: (**a, c**) Urine sediment showing malignant cells with irregular, enlarged and hyperchromatic nuclei and high N:C. The background, however, is different. In the case of carcinoma in situ (**a**) it is clean and the cells are mostly single (SP, ×60). In the case of invasive carcinoma (**c**) background shows marked inflammation and necrosis and cells are single and in loosely cohesive clusters (TP, ×40); (**b, d**) Histology of the two cases (**b**, H&E ×40 and **d**, H&E ×20)

inflammation and necrosis are commonly observed in invasive cancer. Compare the background in carcinoma in situ as seen in Fig. 6.18a with that of invasive carcinoma in Fig. 6.18c.

The high-grade tumors shed cancer cells that are of variable size and configuration with a very high nucleus to cytoplasmic ratio. The nuclei are typically of irregular abnormal shape, although some are approximately spherical or oval. The most important abnormality in urothelial cancer cell is nuclear hyperchromasia caused by abnormal *chromatin texture*: the chromatin is arranged in large, coarse, tightly packed or superimposed granules, sometimes rendering the nucleus dark and nontransparent (India-ink nucleus). Although most cancer cells have a basophilic cytoplasm, the presence of single keratinized cancer cells with eosinophilic cytoplasm is not rare. Figure 6.19a, b is another example of carcinoma in situ. Figure 6.20a–i demonstrates single cells and cell clusters in invasive carcinoma. Compare the malignant cells with nuclei of benign cells, depicting a finely textured "salt-and-pepper" appearance due to small chromatin granules, separated from each other by areas of translucent nucleoplasm (Fig. 6.21a, b). Practically speaking, one can see through a normal nucleus but not through the nucleus of a cancer cell. In liquid-based preparations, this feature is most pronounced in ThinPrep (Fig. 6.20a–f and i). The malignant papillary tumors, even highly anaplastic, may shed cancer cells in large clusters, sometimes reminiscent of papillary arrangement (Fig. 6.22a–c). However, single cancer cells are always present and are usually numerous (Fig. 6.22d). Under these circumstances, it is impossible to determine whether or not a high-grade papillary tumor is invasive. In some advanced

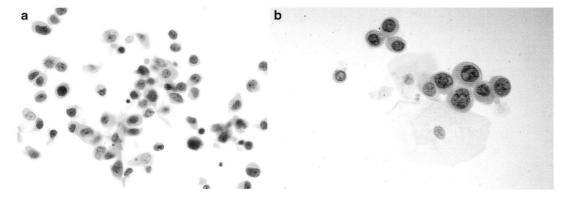

Fig. 6.19 (**a, b**) Urine sediment showing other examples of the clean background and singly dispersed cells in carcinoma in situ (**a**, SP ×40 and **b**, CS ×60)

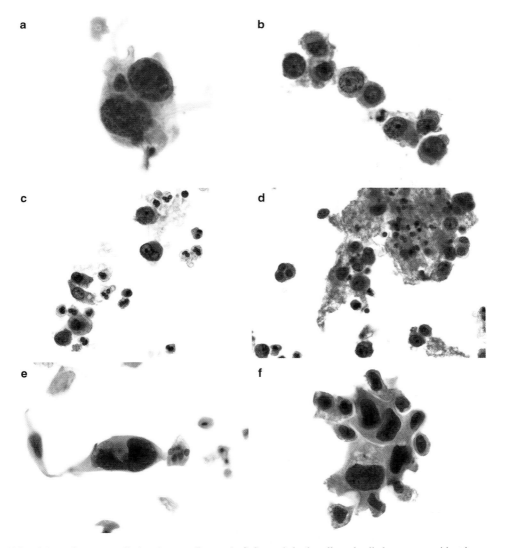

Fig. 6.20 High-grade cancer cells in urinary sediment: (**a–i**) Several single cells and cell clusters are evident in a necrotic background. The cancer cells are variably sized showing large, irregular spherical or oval nucleus, coarsely granulated chromatin and prominent nucleoli and a very high N:C ratio (TP: **a, b, f, i**, ×60 and **c, d, e, g**, ×40 and MF: H ×60). In (**e, f**) the nucleus appears dark & non-transparent due to the coarse chromatin texture (India-ink nucleus)

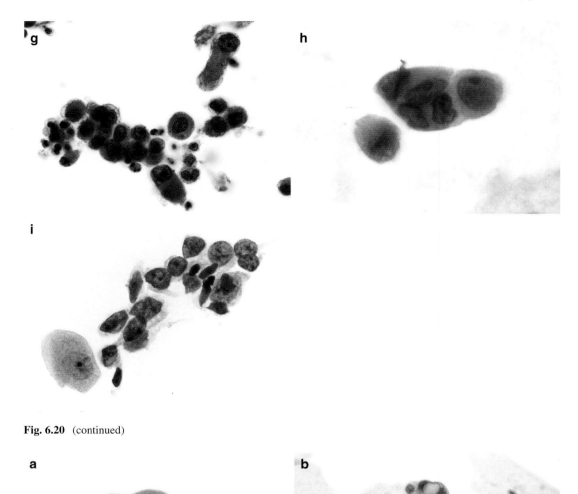

Fig. 6.20 (continued)

Fig. 6.21 (**a**, **b**) Compare benign urothelial cells with finely textured pale chromatin and round uniform nuclei and abundant finely vacuolated cytoplasm with the tumor cells (TP ×60)

cancers with necrotic surface, the yield of cancer cells may be very low. Other features of malignancy include presence of mitoses and lack of umbrella cells. The cytology of high-grade tumors is comparable on ThinPrep and SurePath methods.

It has been shown that in metastatic urothelial carcinoma some cancer cells have a nucleated globular body and a unipolar nontapering cytoplasmic process or "tail." The end of the tail could either be

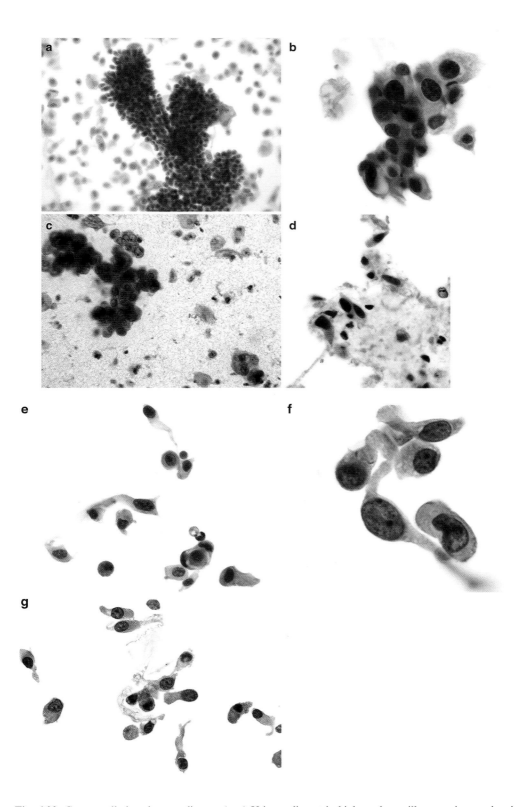

Fig. 6.22 Cancer cells in urinary sediment: (**a–c**) Urine sediment in high-grade papillary carcinoma showing large clusters of cancers, reminiscent of papillary arrangement (SP, ×40, TP, ×60 and MF, ×40); (**d**) However, numerous single cancer cells can be numerous (TP, ×40); (**e**) another example of a high-grade papillary carcinoma in voided urine sediment showing "fish tail" or "cercariform cells." The cells have a globular nucleated body and a unipolar non-tapering cytoplasmic process or "tail"; (**g**) "attempted pearl" formation and "cannibalism" was also be noted in (**e**) (TP: **e**, **g**×40, and **f** ×60)

flattened or bulbous ("fish tail" or "cercariform cells"). The "cercariform" cells may be observed on occasion in urinary sediment of high-grade papillary carcinomas (Fig. 6.22e–g). In addition cell cannibalism and attempted pearl formation may also be noted in these tumors (Fig. 6.22g).

Histologic Variants of Urothelial Carcinoma

Squamous (Keratinizing) Carcinoma

The presence of a focal squamous component in urothelial carcinomas of various types may be seen.

Bladder cancers made up predominantly or exclusively of squamous (keratinizing) cell types are common among patients with *S. haematobium* infestation (see introductory remarks to this chapter and Chap. 5). Rarely, such tumors may originate in areas of squamous metaplasia or leukoplakia, although this cannot always be conclusively documented. Squamous carcinomas, like urothelial carcinomas, may be graded according to the degree of differentiation. The very well-differentiated grade I variety, which may mimic verrucous carcinomas of other organs, is notorious for local growth and late occurrence of metastases. Patients with this type of bladder cancer, particularly common in the presence of Schistosoma, may die of uremia because of obstruction of the ureters by the tumor. Squamous cancers of higher grades are fully capable of metastases and may occur not only in the bladder but also in the ureters and the renal pelves.

The *cytologic presentation* of well-differentiated invasive squamous carcinoma in voided urine is fairly characteristic. In Papanicolaou stain the tumor cells are markedly keratinized with thick, yellow- or orange-colored cytoplasm, and large, irregular, often dark, and pyknotic nuclei (Fig. 6.23a–d). The so-called squamous pearls, cell aggregates concentrically arranged around a core of keratin, may be observed. Anucleated keratin fragments, also known as "ghost cells," are not uncommon. It must be noted that ghost cells may also be derived from benign leukoplakia; such patients should always be investigated further, to rule out squamous carcinoma. Of special interest in the differential diagnosis of well-differentiated squamous carcinomas are the relatively rare condylomata acuminata of the urethra or the bladder that may mimic cytologically squamous cancers (see Fig. 5.11a–c).

Poorly differentiated squamous carcinomas shed in urine a mixture of cancer cells. Some of them show a sharply-demarcated, eosinophilic cytoplasm and large pyknotic nuclei, characteristic of squamous cancer.

Metastatic squamous carcinomas of various primary origins may also occur in the bladder. *In women*, squamous carcinoma of the uterine cervix or vagina that may invade the bladder is of particular importance in this regard. Also in women it is not uncommon to find *squamous cancer cells in the sediment of voided urine that reflect a contamination with cells derived from precancerous lesions of the female genital tract, such as the cervix or vagina*. These events may be suspected if the cancer cells cannot be traced to a bladder lesion. In such instances the investigation of the genital tract is mandatory.

Adenocarcinoma and Its Variants

Primary adenocarcinomas may occur anywhere in the lower urinary tract, but most commonly in the bladder. Risk factors for adenocarcinoma of the urinary tract are: extensive intestinal metaplasia, extrophic bladders, cystitis glandularis, nephrogenic adenoma and villous adenoma that resembles very closely a similar lesion of the colon.

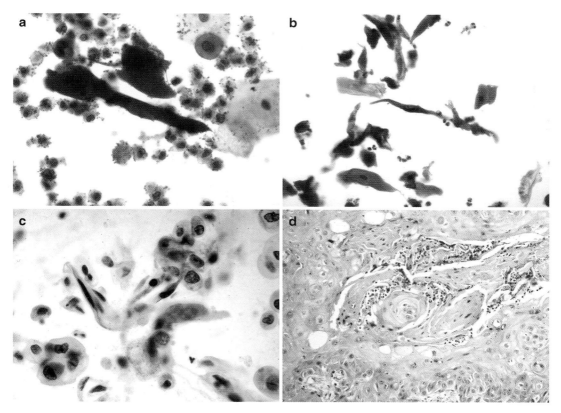

Fig. 6.23 Squamous carcinoma of bladder. Cytologic presentation of this tumor type in the urinary sediment. (**a**, **b**) the sediment shows squamous cells with orangeophilic cytoplasm and opaque, pale nuclei. The pleomorphism of nuclei and the cytoplasm is diagnostic. *Background* shows inflammation (TP ×60 and ×40 resp.); (**c**) Dispersed squamous cancer cells displaying "fiber" cells of squamous carcinoma (CS ×40); (**d**) Squamous carcinoma of the urinary bladder, corresponding to **a** and **b** (H&E ×20)

Adenocarcinoma of the urothelium often closely resembles intestinal carcinomas reflecting the origin of the bladder in the cloaca, the terminal portion of the embryonal intestinal tract (Fig. 6.24a). Tumors derived from the urachus, the vestigial omphalomesenteric duct, usually involve the dome of the bladder. Less common type is mucus-producing signet ring cell carcinoma, infiltrating bladder wall and causing a "leather bottle" bladder, similar to the "leather bottle" stomach (Fig. 6.13b). Other variants of adenocarcinoma include clear cell carcinomas and poorly differentiated adenocarcinomas that may be difficult to classify further.

Cytologically, in classical cases of adenocarcinoma of colonic type the urinary sediment often contains clusters of columnar cancer cells with vacuolated cytoplasm and large nuclei containing nucleoli (Fig. 6.24b, c). In less classical cases, such as the moderately differentiated adenocarcinomas, the cancer cells are more spherical or cuboidal in shape, and are provided with fairly large, hyperchromatic nuclei. Prominent nucleoli may be present. In the presence of large cytoplasmic vacuoles, usually containing mucus, the nuclei may be pushed to the periphery of the cell (signet-ring cells) (Fig. 6.24d, e). In the poorly differentiated tumors, the type of tumor cannot be established on cytologic grounds. In clear cell adenocarcinoma the cancer cells are usually quite large, have an abundant, faintly granular or finely vacuolated cytoplasm and open, vesicular nuclei with prominent nucleoli (Fig. 6.24f).

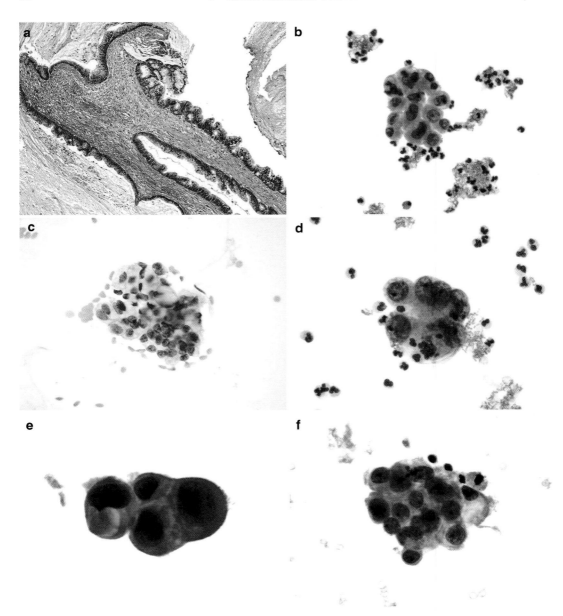

Fig. 6.24 Adenocarcinoma of bladder. (**a**) Histology of urachal adenocarcinoma resembling intestinal carcinoma (H&E ×10); (**b, c**) Corresponding voided urine sediment shows a cluster of cancer cells with vacuolated cytoplasm and hyperchromatic rounded nuclei with prominent nucleoli (TP ×60); (**d, e**) Examples of moderately differentiated adenocarcinoma showing cancer cells with large spherical nuclei and prominent nucleoli. Large cytoplasmic vacuoles displace the nucleus peripherally (TP ×60); (**f**) Clear cell adenocarcinoma in voided urine sediment (TP ×60)

The differential diagnosis of primary adenocarcinoma of the bladder comprises metastatic adenocarcinomas of various origins, particularly of the rectum or colon that have a very similar histologic and cytologic makeup (see below).

Small Cell (Oat Cell) Carcinomas

Small cell carcinomas (oat cell carcinomas) of the bladder are highly malignant and very aggressive tumors, similar in appearance and behavior to tumors of the lung and other organs. The neuroendocrine nature of these tumors may require immunostaining. The cancer cells are small, larger than lymphocytes, and are characterized by compact, often pyknotic nuclei and very scanty, usually basophilic cytoplasm. There are no visible nucleoli. Of diagnostic significance in cytologic presentation of oat cell carcinoma is the presence of small clusters or rouleaux of tightly packed tumor cells with nuclear molding (Figs. 6.25 and 6.26). The absence of nucleoli and the presence of cell clusters are very helpful in differentiating the cells of oat cell carcinoma from a malignant lymphoma wherein the cells, as a rule, do not cluster and are usually provided with nucleoli (see below). However, in the currently used liquid-based preparations the classic features of small cell carcinoma may be altered. Single cells may be numerous, cells may show less nuclear molding and crush artifact and nucleoli and cytoplasm may be more readily observed.

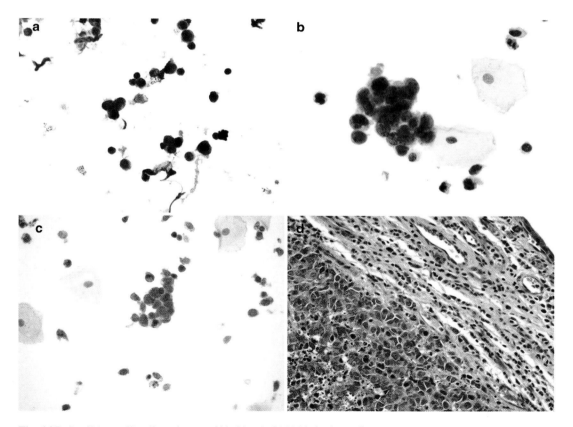

Fig. 6.25 Small (oat cell) cell carcinoma of bladder. (**a, b**) Voided urine sediment shows small cancer cells, larger than lymphocytes, with compact pyknotic nuclei and very scanty, basophilic cytoplasm. There are no visible nucleoli (TP ×40 and ×60); (**c**) Positive synpatophysin in ThinPrep (×60); (**d**) corresponding histology of small cell carcinoma in bladder biopsy (H&E ×40)

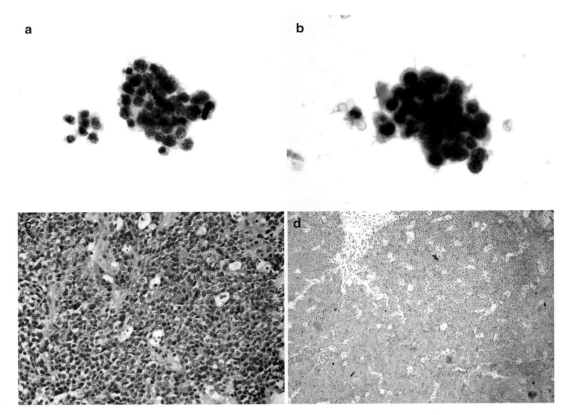

Fig. 6.26 Another example of small (oat cell) cell carcinoma of bladder. (**a, b**) In ThinPrep, cytoplasm and nucleoli may be evident and nuclear molding and crush artifact are less pronounced (TP ×60); (**c, d**) corresponding histology and positive synpatophysin (H&E ×40)

Other rare primary tumors include spindle and giant cell carcinomas, mesodermal mixed tumors, lymphoepithelioma-like carcinomas, sarcomas, multiple myeloma, choriocarcinoma, malignant lymphoma, and primary melanoma. The latter two are discussed below with metastatic tumors. For other rare primary tumors of the bladder consult the references cited and also see Koss's Diagnostic Cytology and Its Histopathologic Bases. 5th Ed, pp. 813–816.

Metastatic Tumors

A broad spectrum of metastatic malignant tumors may also be observed in the urinary sediment. By far the most common metastatic tumors are derived from adjacent organs: in women the uterine cervix or sometimes the endometrium and ovary; in men the prostate, and in both sexes the colon and rectum. Distant metastasis of mammary carcinoma is not uncommon in women.

Carcinoma and Precancerous States of the Uterine Cervix

This is an important source of abnormal cells in the urinary sediment. In invasive cancer the cancer cells may desquamate directly into the lumen of the urinary bladder. In precancerous states the cells

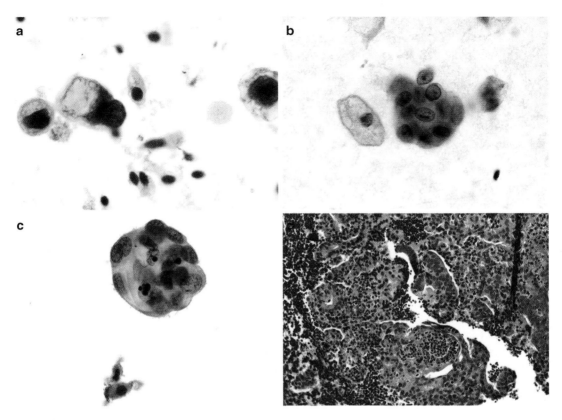

Fig. 6.27 Metastatic carcinoma to the urinary tract. (**a**, **b**) Two examples of metastatic ovarian carcinoma to the urinary tract (**a**, CS ×40; **b**, MF ×60). Note the large cells with clear cytoplasm and cluster of much smaller cells corresponding to ovarian tumor; (**c**) metastatic endometrial carcinoma (TP ×60); (**d**) histology of endometrial primary (H&E ×10)

desquamating from the surface of the cervix may be picked up by the urinary stream. In both situations the cells have the characteristics of a squamous carcinoma as seen in Papanicolaou stain. If such cells are found in the urinary sediment of women in the absence of a documented primary bladder carcinoma, it is advisable to have these patients investigated by means of a cervical smear and a colposcopic examination of the uterine cervix.

Other Carcinomas of the Female Genital Tract

Ovarian and endometrial adenocarcinomas may invade the wall of the urinary bladder and may display in the urinary sediment single cancer cells or, more commonly, cell clusters, characteristic of these diseases. The cancer cells are usually quite large, often larger in ovarian than endometrial cancer, and are characterized by a basophilic, often vacuolated cytoplasm and open, vesicular, large nuclei, provided with large nucleoli. Such cells cannot be differentiated from cells of some types of a primary adenocarcinoma of the bladder, except on clinical grounds and by histologic examination (Fig. 6.27a–d).

Fig. 6.28 Metastatic tumors
to the urinary tract. Example
of colonic carcinoma
metastasis (TP ×40)

Prostatic Carcinoma

Usually in advanced stages of the disease, prostatic adenocarcinoma may invade the urinary bladder or metastasize to it. The cancer cells in the urinary sediment are usually quite small, often spherical, but sometimes columnar in configuration. The cells often occur singly but may form clusters. The principal feature of these cells is the presence of delicate and prominent nucleoli. Immunostaining for racemase, prostatic specific antigen or prostatic alkaline phosphatase allows their identification. Still, it must be stressed that some bladder tumors originating in the trigone may share the immune characteristics with prostatic cells. Therefore, the knowledge of clinical history is essential. Another important point in the differential diagnosis of prostatic carcinoma is the synchronous presence of prostatic and bladder tumors, as extensively documented by mapping studies (Mahadevia et al.). Thus it is not uncommon to observe urothelial carcinomas, sometimes as flat carcinomas in situ, accompanying prostatic disease.

Carcinomas of Colon and Rectum

Cells of colorectal carcinoma are a frequent finding in urinary sediment and may be the result of direct extension of rectal cancer to the urinary tract or metastasis from a distant portion of the bowel. The columnar cells of metastatic colonic carcinoma may be similar to primary adenocarcinoma of the urinary bladder. Tumor identification is aided by clinical and histologic examination and immunocytochemical stain results (Fig. 6.28). Tumors of colonic origin stain positive for CK20 and CDX-2, while primary bladder adenocarcinoma is negative for CDX-2.

Carcinoma of Renal Cell Origin

Rarely, renal cell carcinoma may metastasize or be present in voided urine cytology (Fig. 6.29a–d). Cancer cells are usually large with clear or vacuolated cytoplasm, round nucleus with prominent nucleolus. Immunostains may be helpful.

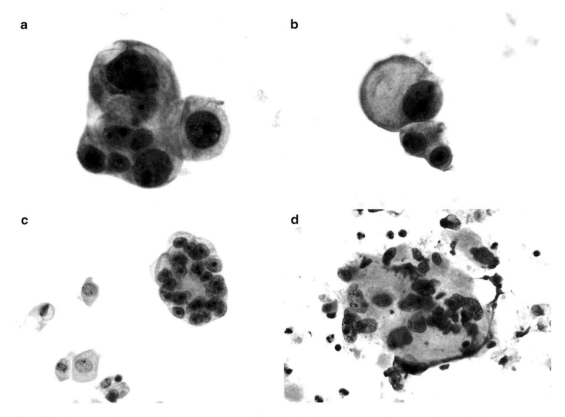

Fig. 6.29 Metastatic tumors to the urinary tract. (**a–c**) Voided urine sediment with metastatic renal cell carcinoma to the bladder (TP ×60); (**d**) direct smear from fine needle aspiration of liver metastasis from this case (×60)

Metastatic Carcinomas from Distant Sites

Occasionally, carcinomas from more distant primary sites may be observed in the urinary sediment. In women, by far the most common such cancers are of mammary origin. In men the most common source of metastatic carcinoma is lung cancer. It is usually not possible to distinguish primary bladder from a metastasis on cytologic grounds with the exception of tumors of hematopoietic system and malignant melanoma.

Other Metastatic Tumors

Malignant lymphoma and leukemia are one of the important sources of metastatic disease. Non-Hodgkin's lymphomas, particularly of the large cell type, may be identified in the sediment of voided urine. The tumors cells usually appear singly and do not form clusters, have scanty cytoplasm, and show significant nuclear abnormalities of various types. Thus the nuclei may be of bizarre shapes or show the characteristic nuclear protrusions or "nipples." In other cells the nuclei may be indented or cleaved. Prominent nucleoli, sometimes multiple, are commonly observed. Non-Hodgkin's lymphomas may have a variety of cytologic presentations, depending on tumor type, and the reader is referred to other sources for a detailed analysis (Fig. 6.30a, b).

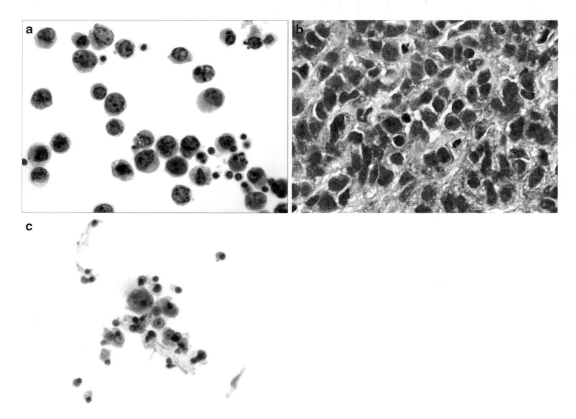

Fig. 6.30 Metastatic tumors to the urinary tract. (**a**) Example of malignant lymphoma metastatic to bladder. Note atypical lymphoid cells (TP ×40); (**b**) Corresponding biopsy (H&E ×40); (**c**) Metastatic melanoma. Note pigmented cancer cells in urine sediment (TP ×40)

Metastatic malignant melanoma may involve the urinary tract. Melanoma may be associated with melanuria that indicates that the kidney may also be involved by the tumor. Cells of malignant melanoma are characterized by significant abnormalities in cell size, configuration, and nuclear structure. In most instances the cancer cells are large, sometimes very large, containing one, two or sometimes more nuclei, often located at the periphery of the cell, with very large nucleoli and intranuclear cytoplasmic inclusions. The cytoplasm of the tumor cells usually contains abundant brown melanin pigment (Fig. 6.30c). It is not possible to determine from the positive urinary sediment which part of the urinary tract is involved by tumor, which may affect the kidneys, the ureters, or the bladder, sometimes all sites at once. The very uncommon primary melonomas of the baldder have an identical cytologic presentation.

Cytologic Monitoring of Patients Treated for Tumors of Lower Urinary Tract

Cytologic monitoring of patients treated for tumors of the lower urinary tract is effective only in early detection of new or recurrent high-grade tumors. Urinary tract cytology has so far not replaced cystoscopy in the follow-up and identification of low-grade papillary tumors. In our experience, the best method of monitoring bladder tumors is by cytologic analysis of voided urine specimens. After radical cystectomy, the patients must be monitored by periodic cytologic examination of urine from the ileal bladder. The monitoring may be required for many years after treatment. Patients treated for carcinoma of the renal pelvis and ureter who are also prone to the development of new carcinomas elsewhere in the urinary tract, should also be monitored by urinary cytology.

Each monitoring sequence should be based on three urine samples obtained on consecutive days. The presence of cancer cells, as described in the preceding pages, is always indicative of a recurrence or progression of urothelial carcinoma, regardless of the mode of treatment or presumed clinical status. Cytologic analysis is more sensitive than multiple biopsies in predicting tumor recurrence or progression. Patients with seemingly innocuous low-grade tumors may develop an unexpected invasive cancer of the bladder, presumably derived from adjacent carcinoma in situ and related lesions.

None of the cytotoxic drugs or BCG causes epithelial cell changes that could be confused with cancer. Although minor atypias in the form of cellular and nuclear enlargement may be observed with thiotepa, neither mitomycin nor BCG causes any significant cytologic abnormalities, except for granulomatous inflammation in BCG. The granulomas may be observed in the urinary sediment, as described in Chap. 5.

Monitoring of patients undergoing radiotherapy is difficult because of radiation changes affecting benign epithelial cells, as discussed in Chap. 5. Radiotherapy of carcinomas of the bladder may cause nuclear pyknosis and ballooning of the tumor cells, a change often reflected in urinary sediment. The degree of nuclear abnormality in the cancer cells usually, but not always, allows a differentiation between the irradiated benign and the irradiated malignant cells. However, when the nuclei of irradiated benign cells show nuclear hyperchromasia, the differential diagnosis becomes difficult. In such situations, it is advisable to withhold judgment until clear-cut evidence of cancer is obtained on subsequent samples of urine. The cells of bladder cancer recurring after radiotherapy are in no way different from the cells of the primary tumor. Numerous biopsies may often be required to obtain histologic confirmation of a tumor, especially if there is considerable scarring of the bladder wall.

As emphasized above, the cytologic approach to monitoring of treated patients will fail in discovering new or recurrent low-grade papillary tumors. This fundamental fact has led to the development of a substantial number of new methods of monitoring of bladder tumors (see Chap. 7).

Reporting of Cytologic Findings

Translation of cytologic diagnostic categories into surgical pathology diagnoses is a difficult and complicated matter. Moreover, there is no consensus on diagnostic terminologies for urothelial cytology. Currently, the following categories are commonly utilized: negative, atypical, suspicious, and positive for malignant cells. The cytologic features that are evaluated include background, cellularity, cell arrangement, nuclear and cytoplasmic features. The architectural features include fibrovascular cores and cellular organization and crowding. These features have been addressed for benign entities (negative) in Chap. 5 and for neoplastic lesions (suspicious and positive) in this chapter.

The term "atypia" is commonly used when morphologic changes exceed those seen in benign entities but lack clear neoplastic changes. However, this term is of very little value to the clinicians and should be avoided whenever possible. The recognition of exact nature of "atypical cells" in urine is a major challenge for cytopathologists. Atypical cells belong to two categories: those corresponding to benign conditions, and those reflecting urothelial tumors. Unfortunately, in daily microscopic work these fine points of differentiation cannot be recognized. Further subdividing atypical cases into the categories of "favor reactive" and "atypia of undetermined significance" does not add clinically relevant information. It may be of value to consider the possibility of reactive cellular changes or artifacts whenever atypia is encountered on urine cytology. Conceivably the reporting of findings showing or not showing cancer cells is easy to implement.

Benign conditions that are important source of error include lithiasis, instrumentation, polyomavirus infection, or treatment effect (Figs. 4.6, 5.9, 5.15, and 5.18). Urothelial tumors leading to an atypical diagnosis predominantly include low-grade papillary tumors (Figs. 6.9 and 6.10).

In some cases the separation of "atypical" from "suspicious" or outright malignant cells may become a matter for a debate that is not easily settled. In such cases, it is important to secure a patient's history and cystoscopic findings before formulating a clinical recommendation. Usually, the significance of the "atypical" cells will be fairly easily determined. Still, in some cases, long-term follow-up and multiple bladder biopsies may be required to rule out a neoplastic process.

Key Points

- The most important accomplishment of cytology of the urinary tract is the diagnosis of clinically unsuspected cases of high-grade urothelial carcinoma in situ and invasive carcinoma.
- Cytologic monitoring of patients treated for tumors of the lower urinary tract is effective only in early detection of new or recurrent high-grade tumors. The success of cytologic monitoring depends greatly on the type of tumor and the mode of therapy.
- Voided urine has an excellent diagnostic performance for high-grade tumors, particularly carcinoma in situ and invasive cancers.
- Failures to establish a cytologic diagnosis are mainly with low-grade urothelial tumors.
- Cytologic monitoring of patients treated for tumors of the lower urinary tract is effective only in early detection of new or recurrent high-grade tumors. Urinary tract cytology has so far not replaced cystoscopy in the follow-up and identification of new low-grade papillary bladder tumors.
- None of the cytotoxic drugs or BCG causes epithelial cell changes that could be confused with cancer.
- The degree of nuclear abnormality in irradiated malignant cells allows a differentiation from irradiated benign cells.
- Since cytologic approach to monitoring of treated patients may fail to detect new or recurrent low-grade papillary tumors, which has led to the development of a substantial number of new non-cytologic methods of monitoring of bladder tumors.
- *It must be clearly understood that the diagnosis of cancer rendered by a competent observer on multiple urine samples must be taken with utmost seriousness. This usually indicates the presence of a life-threatening disease. It must be remembered that invasive cancer is in most instances not associated with visible, papillary disease but with the invisible carcinoma in situ and that ignoring a positive cytologic report may lead to a disaster for the patient. It is of additional significance that patients undergoing local chemotherapy, whether by thiotepa, mitamycin C, or bacillus calmette-guerin (BCG) are not exempt from this rule. The presence of cancer cells in the sediment indicates treatment failure. It is rare for the drug effect to be confused with cancer.*

Suggested Readings

1. Acs G, Gupta PK, Baloch ZW. Cytomorphology of high-grade neuroenedocrine carcinoma of the urinary tract. Diagn Cytopathol. 2000;23:92–6.
2. Alsheikh A, Mohamedali Z, Jones E, et al. Comparison of the WHO/ISUP classification and cyctokeratin 20 expression in predicting the behavior of low-grade papillary urothelial tumors. World/Health Organization/International Society of Urologic Pathology. Mod Pathol. 2001;14:267–72.
3. Renshaw AA. Atypical urinary cytology specimens. Cancer Cytopathol. 2000;90:222–9.

4. Banigo OG, Waisman J, Kaufman JJ. Papillary (transitional) carcinoma in an ileal conduit. J Urol. 1975;114:626–7.
5. Bardales RH, Pitman MB, Stanley MW, et al. Urine cytology of primary and secondary urinary bladder adenocarcinoma. Cancer. 1998;84:335–43.
6. Bastacky S, Ibrahim S, Wilczynski SP, et al. The accuracy of urinary cytology in daily practice. Cancer. 1999; 87:118–28.
7. Boon ME, Blomjous CE, Zwartendijk J, et al. Carcinoma in situ of the urinary bladder. Clinical presentation, cytologic pattern and stromal changes. Acta Cytol. 1986;30:360–6.
8. Brosman SA. The use of bacillus Calmette-Guerin in the therapy of bladder carcinoma in situ. J Urol. 1985;134:36–9.
9. Cecchini S, Cipparrone I, Confortini M, et al. Urethral cytology of Cytobrush specimens. A new technique for detecting subclinical human papillomavirus infection in men. Acta Cytol. 1988;32:314–7.
10. Chan TY, Epstein JI. In situ adenocarcinoma of the bladder. Am J Surg Pathol. 2001;25:892–9.
11. Cheng L, Cheville JC, Neumann RM, et al. Survival of patients with carcinoma in situ of the urinary bladder. Cancer. 1999;85:2469–74.
12. Cheng L, Cheville JC, Neumann RM, et al. Flat intraepithelial lesions of the urinary bladder. Cancer. 2000; 88:625–31.
13. Cheng L, Darson M, Cheville JC, et al. Urothelial papilloma of the bladder. Clinical and biological implications. Cancer. 1999;86:2098–101.
14. Cheng L, Neumann RM, Bostwick DG. Papillary urothelial neoplasms of low malignant potential. Clinical and biological implications. Cancer. 1999;86:2102–8.
15. Czerniak B, Koss LG, Sherman A. Nuclear pores and DNA ploidy in human bladder carcinomas. Cancer Res. 1984;44:3752–6.
16. Czerniak B, Koss LG. Expression of Ca antigen on human urinary bladder tumors. Cancer. 1985;55:2380–3.
17. Cina SJ, Lancaster-Weiss KJ, Lecksell K, et al. Correlation of Ki-67 and p53 with the new World Health Organization/International Society of Urological Pathology Classification System for Urothelial Noeplasia. Arch Pathol Lab Med. 2001;125:646–51.
18. Crosby JH, Allsbrook Jr WC, Koss LG, et al. Cytologic detection of urothelial cancer and other abnormalities in a cohort of workers exposed to aromatic amines. Acta Cytol. 1991;35:263–8.
19. Curry JL, Wojcik EM. The effects of the current World Health Organization/International Society of Urologic Pathologists bladder neoplasm classification system on urine cytology results. Cancer. 2002;96:140–5.
20. Deshpande V, McKee GT. Analysis of atypical urine cytology in a tertiary care center. Cancer. 2005;105: 468–75.
21. Eble JN, Sauter G, Epstein JI, et al. World health organization classification of tumours. In: Pathology and genetics of tumours of the urinary system and male genital organs. Lyon, France: IARC Press; 2004.
22. Epstein JI, Amin MB, Reuter VR, et al. The World Health Organization/International Society of Urological Pathology consensus classification of urothelial (transitional cell) neoplasms of the urinary bladder. Bladder Consensus Conference Committee. Am J Surg Pathol. 1998;22:1435–48.
23. Epstein JI. Diagnosis and classification of flat, papillary, and invasive urothelial carcinoma: the WHO/ISUP consensus. Int J Surg Pathol. 2010;18:106S–11. Review.
24. Genega EM, Porter CR. Urothelial neoplasms of the kidney and ureter. An epidemiologic, pathologic, and clinical review. Am J Clin Pathol. 2002;117:S36–48. Review.
25. Glatz K, Willi N, Glatz D, et al. An international telecytologic quiz on urinary cytology reveals educational deficits and absence of a commonly used classification system. Am J Clin Pathol. 2006;126:294–301.
26. Goldstein ML, Whitman T, Renshaw AA. Significance of cell groups in voided urine. Acta Cytol. 1998;42: 290–4.
27. Grignon DJ, Ro JY, Ayala AG, et al. Primary adenocarcinoma of the urinary bladder. A clinicopathologic analysis of 72 cases. Cancer. 1991;67:2165–72.
28. Grignon DJ, Ro JY, Ayala AG, et al. Small cell carcinoma of the urinary bladder. A clinicopathologic analysis of 22 cases. Cancer. 1992;69:527–36.
29. Herawi M, Parwani AV, Chan T, et al. Polyoma virus-associated cellular changes in the urine and bladder biopsy samples: a cytohistologic correlation. Am J Surg Pathol. 2006;30:345–50.
30. Hughes JH, Raab SS, Cohen MB. The cytologic diagnosis of low-grade transitional cell carcinoma. Am J Clin Pathol. 2000;114:S59–67. Review.
31. Jemal A, Siegel R, Xu J, et al. Cancer statistics, 2010. CA Cancer J Clin. 2010;60:277–300.
32. Kannan V, Bose S. Low grade transitional cell carcinoma and instrument artifact. A challenge in urinary cytology. Acta Cytol. 1993;37:899–902.
33. Kapur U, Venkataraman G, Wojcik EM. Diagnostic significance of 'atypia' in instrumented versus voided urine specimens. Cancer Cytopathol. 2008;114:270–4.
34. Koss LG. Mapping of the urinary bladder: its impact on the concepts of bladder cancer. Hum Pathol. 1979; 10:533–48.

35. Koss LG. Evaluation of patients with carcinoma in situ of the bladder. Pathol Annu. 1982;17:353–9.
36. Koss LG, Deitch D, Ramanathan R, et al. Diagnostic value of cytology of voided urine. Acta Cytol. 1985;29: 810–6.
37. Koss LG. Precursor lesions of invasive bladder cancer. Eur Urol. 1988;14:4–6.
38. Koss LG. Tumors of the urinary tract in urine and brushings. In: Koss LG, Melamed MR, editors. Koss's diagnostic cytology and its histopathologic bases. 5th ed. Philadelphia, PA: Lippincott Williams & Wilkins; 2006. p. 777–846.
39. Krishnan B, Truong LD. Prostatic adenocarcinoma diagnosed by urinary cytology. Am J Clin Pathol. 2000;113:29–34.
40. Melicow MM, Hollowell JW. Intra-urothelial cancer: carcinoma in situ, Bowen's disease of the urinary system: discussion of thirty cases. J Urol. 1952;68:763–72.
41. Murphy WM, Soloway MS, Jukkola AF, et al. Urinary cytology and bladder cancer. The cellular features of transitional cell neoplasms. Cancer. 1984;53:1555–65.
42. Nasuti JF, Fleisher SR, et al. Significance of tissue fragments in voided urine specimens. Acta Cytol. 2001;45: 147–52.
43. Pich A, Chiusa L, Formiconi A, et al. Biologic differences between noninvasive papillary urothelial neoplasms of low malignant potential and low-grade (grade 1) papillary carcinomas of the bladder. Am J Surg Pathol. 2001; 25:1528–33.
44. Raab SS, Lenel JC, Cohen MB. Low grade transitional cell carcinoma of the bladder. Cytologic diagnosis by key features as identified by logistic regression analysis. Cancer. 1994;74:1621–6.
45. Raab SS, Grzybicki DM, Vrbin CM, et al. Urine cytology discrepancies: frequency, causes, and outcomes. Am J Clin Pathol. 2007;127:946–53.
46. Renshaw AA, Nappi D, Weinberg DS. Cytology of grade 1 papillary transitional cell carcinoma. A comparison of cytologic, architectural and morphometric criteria in cystoscopically obtained urine. Acta Cytol. 1996;40:676–82.
47. Richter J, Jiang F, Görög JP, et al. Marked genetic differences between stage pTa and stage pT1 papillary bladder cancer detected by comparative genomic hybridization. Cancer Res. 1997;57:2860–4.
48. Rosenthal DL, Raab SS. Cytologic detection of urothelial lesions. New York, NY: Springer; 2006. p. 57–120.
49. Taylor DC, Bhagavan BS, Larsen MP, et al. Papillary urothelial hyperplasia. A precursor to papillary neoplasms. Am J Surg Pathol. 1996;20:1481–8.
50. Trillo AA, Kuchler LL, Wood AC, et al. Adenocarcinoma of the urinary bladder: histologic, cytologic and ultrastructural features in a case. Acta Cytol. 1981;25:285–90.
51. Van Hoeven KH, Artymyshyn RL. Cytology of small cell carcinoma of the urinary bladder. Diagn Cytopathol. 1996;14:292–7.
52. Weaver EJ, McCue PA, Bagley DH, et al. Expression of cytokeratin 20 and CD44 protein in upper urinary tract transitional cell carcinoma: cytologic-histologic correlation. Anal Quant Cytol Histol. 2001;23:339–44.
53. Witte D, Truong LD, Ramzy I. Transitional cell carcinoma of the renal pelvis the diagnostic role of pelvic washings. Am J Clin Pathol. 2002;117:444–50.
54. Wojcik EM, Brownlie RJ, Bassler TJ, et al. Superficial urothelial (umbrella) cells. A potential cause of abnormal DNA ploidy results in urine specimens. Anal Quant Cytol Histol. 2000;22:411–5.
55. Wojcik EM, Saraga SA, Jin JK, et al. Application of laser scanning cytometry for evaluation of DNA ploidy in routine cytologic specimens. Diagn Cytopathol. 2001;24:200–5.
56. Xin W, Raab SS, Michael CW. Low-grade urothelial carcinoma: reappraisal of the cytologic criteria on ThinPrep. Diagn Cytopathol. 2003;29:125–9.
57. Young RH. Carcinosarcoma of the urinary bladder. Cancer. 1987;59:1333–9.

Chapter 7
Urine-Based Assays Complementing Cytologic Examination in the Detection of Urothelial Neoplasm

Hiroshi Miyamoto

Keywords US FDA-approved markers • Bladder tumor antigen • Nuclear matrix protein 22 • Fibrin–fibrinogen degradation product • ImmunoCyt • UroVysion • Bladder cancer antigen • Survivin • UBC tests • CYFRA 21-1 • Hyaluronic acid-hyaluronidase • Telomerase • Quanticyt • Fibroblast growth factor receptor 3 • Mucin 7 • MUC7 • VEGF • Immunocytochemistry • Cytokeratins • p53 • Ki-67 • p16 • EGFR • E-cadherin • DD23

Introduction

In this chapter, five markers of bladder cancer approved by the US Food and Drug Administration (FDA), as well as ten other urine-based markers that have been shown to be clinically useful, all of which could be substitutes of cystoscopy and/or cytology. Immunocytochemical detection of markers in exfoliated urothelial cells is separately reviewed. Comparison of urine markers and cytology as to the sensitivity, specificity, and cost is also discussed.

US FDA-Approved Markers

Bladder Tumor Antigen (BTA)

Invasive bladder cancer degrades the basement membrane of the extracellular matrix and the specific degradation product can be found in urine. The original BTA test, a qualitative latex agglutination assay that detects these basement membrane antigens, was taken off the market and has been replaced by two test kits approved by the FDA in 1998 for urothelial carcinoma surveillance, in combination with cystoscopy. The BTA-stat® (Polymedco, Cortlandt Manor, New York), a qualitative point-of-care (POC) test, and the BTA-TRAK® (Polymedco), a quantitative enzyme-linked immunosorbent (ELISA) assay, both detect and measure the complement factor H and its related protein in the urine (Fig. 7.1).

The BTA-stat is an immunoassay performed by placing five drops of urine (stored at room temperature for up to 48 h, at 2–8°C for up to 7 days, or at ≤−20°C for up to 24 weeks) in the sample well of the device and allowing it to react with the antibody for exactly 5 min. A visible pink or reddish-brown line in the test window indicates a positive result, while a line in the control zone assures that the device is working properly. The BTA-TRAK is a standard sandwich immunoassay, using 96-well format, which delivers quantitative results in 2.5 h.

L.G. Koss and R.S. Hoda, *Koss's Cytology of the Urinary Tract with Histopathologic Correlations*, DOI 10.1007/978-1-4614-2056-9_7, © Leopold G. Koss 2012

Fig. 7.1 BTA tests
(Polymedco). BTA-stat®, a
qualitative POC test kit, and
BTA-TRAK®, a quantitative
ELISA assay kit

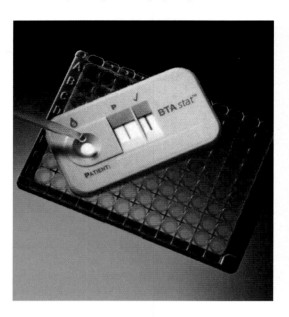

The overall sensitivity of these two tests reported in cohort and case–control studies ranges from 36 to 89% [1–3]. As observed in urine cytology, the sensitivity of BTA tests is dependent on tumor grade, stage, and size, and is lower for detecting low-grade and/or small tumors. Nonetheless, studies have suggested the usefulness of these tests in monitoring disease aggressiveness and predicting tumor recurrence. The specificity of the BTA tests in healthy individuals has been reported to be as high as 97%. However, in patients with various genitourinary conditions including infection, inflammation, calculi, hematuria, and proteinuria, the specificity drops to as low as 46%. In particular, the BTA tests might show a false positivity in conditions causing hematuria due to the presence of complement factor H in human serum at high concentrations (approximately 0.5 mg/mL). In addition, a significant decrease in the specificity in patients who received intravesical instillations (e.g., BCG, mitomycin C) for preventing tumor progression or recurrence was reported. The manufacturer recommends that the BTA-stat and BTA-TRAK tests should be used only in conjunction with information available from the clinical evaluation of the patient and other diagnostic procedures and should not be used as a screening test for individuals without biopsy confirmed bladder cancer.

Nuclear Matrix Protein 22 (NMP22)

NMP22 is a family member of NMPs that are involved in DNA configuration, structure, and function regulating DNA replication, transcription, and gene expression. The NMP22 tests detect a part of nuclear mitotic apparatus protein released from urothelial cells upon cellular apoptosis. Substantially higher levels of NMP22 are detected in the urine from patients with urothelial cancer than in that from healthy individuals. However, urinary NMP22 could be elevated in a number of benign genitourinary conditions, such as urolithiasis, infection, and inflammation, in which increased cell death is present, resulting in a false-positive result. The standard NMP22 test, a quantitative sandwich ELISA, was FDA-approved in 1996 and the qualitative POC assay (BladderChek®; Matritech, Newton, Massachusetts) was approved for prescription use and exempt from Clinical Laboratory Improvement Amendments regulations, as an adjunct to cystoscopy, but not as a stand-alone test, in 2002. The NMP22 BladderChek is performed by applying four drops of fresh (<2 h) voided urine to the sample well of the device and reading test result at 30–50 min after the sample application.

In terms of clinical development, NMP22 is one of the most mature urine markers currently available. Lokeshwar et al. [3] summarized various studies that evaluate NMP22, showing the sensitivity of 47–100%, most often ranging between 60 and 70%, and the specificity of 55–90%, depending on the cutoff value used. Then, two major prospective multicenter (23 clinical sites) clinical trials, using the NMP22 BladderCheck test, were published in the *Journal of American Medical Association* [4, 5].

The first article evaluated the NMP22 POC assay for primary detection involving 1,331 patients with risk factors for bladder cancer (e.g., hematuria, dysuria, history of smoking) [4]. Among 223 patients with a positive test result, 44 were found to have bladder cancer, whereas among 1,108 patients with a negative result, 35 had bladder cancer. Overall sensitivity and specificity of the NMP22 test were 56% and 86%, respectively. The sensitivity in invasive (90%) or high-grade (72%) tumors was higher than that in non-invasive (50%) or low-grade (48%) tumors, respectively. In contrast, cytology performed poorly with an overall sensitivity of 16% (17% in non-invasive vs. 22% in invasive and 0% in low-grade vs. 38% in high-grade tumors). However, overall specificity was still higher for cytology at 99%. In addition, the authors emphasize that the NMP22 test detected four cancers that were not visualized during initial cystoscopy and in which two of them were positive for cytology.

This assay was subsequently evaluated for surveillance for recurrence [5]. Of 668 patients with a history of bladder cancer, 123 positive and 545 negative test results were detected, and 103 (51 with positive and 72 with negative results) developed recurrent tumor. Overall sensitivity and specificity of the NMP22 test were 50% and 87%, respectively. The sensitivity in invasive (91%) or high-grade (75%) tumors was higher than that in non-invasive (44%) or low-grade (39%) tumors, respectively. Although cytology results were not available in five cases in this study, overall sensitivity of cytology was 12% (0% in non-invasive vs. 11% in invasive and 5% in low-grade vs. 19% in high-grade tumors). The authors emphasize that among nine initial cystoscopy-negative cases the NMP22 test detected eight cases whereas cytology did only three cases.

Thus, in the above two studies, the NMP22 POC assay was more significantly sensitive than cytology, although these studies were criticized because of markedly low overall sensitivity for urine cytology compared to previously published data mostly from a single clinical site. More recently, NMP22 positivity prior to the initial resection was shown to have predictive value for future tumor recurrence in patients with high-risk superficial bladder cancer.

Fibrin–Fibrinogen Degradation Product (FDP)

Vascular permeability is often increased in bladder cancer via its production of vascular endothelial growth factor (VEGF). This results in the leakage of plasma proteins, including fibrinogen and plasminogen, into the urine. Subsequently, fibrin converted from fibrinogen is degraded to FDP by plasmin converted from plasminogen. Therefore, patients with bladder cancer could have increased levels of FDP in their urine. AccuDx™ (Intracel, Frederick, Maryland) is a rapid POC immunoassay that detects fibrin-FDP. The sensitivity and specificity of the AccuDx test ranged from 47 to 68% and 25 to 80%, respectively [6]. This test yields higher positive rates, with higher tumor grades and stages, but may also show false positive result particularly in patients with hematuria of various etiologies. The data thus suggested little additional value over cytology for detecting bladder cancer.

ImmunoCyt

ImmunoCyt/uCyt+™ (DiagnoCure, Quebec City, Quebec, Canada) is a cell-based test, combining urinary cytology and fluorescence immunocytochemistry, using three monoclonal antibodies against two bladder cancer-associated mucin glycoproteins and a bladder cancer variant of carcinoembryonic

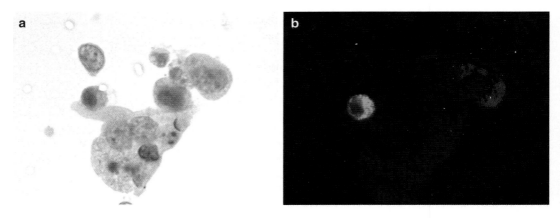

Fig. 7.2 ImmunoCyt™ (DiagnoCure). A combined test with urine cytology (**a**) and fluorescence immunocytochemistry (**b**), using antibodies against mucin antigens (*green*) and CEA antigen (*red*)

antigen (CEA). Specific technical requirements for the ImmunoCyt test include a fluorescence microscope and a cytocentrifuge, and it is, therefore, performed in a reference laboratory. The test is scored as positive when either one green (mucin antigens) or one red (CEA antigen) fluorescence urothelial cell among at least 500 epithelial cells on a slide is identified (Fig. 7.2). False-positive results can be obtained in the presence of prostate cancer cells and a small portion of umbrella cells or normal squamous cells. However, the test is least likely affected by benign genitourinary conditions. There are FDA approval limits of the ImmunoCyt that include use in conjunction with conventional cytology.

The sensitivity and specificity of the ImmunoCyt have been reported to range between 38 and 100% and between 62 and 90%, respectively [2, 3, 7, 8]. The most recent multicenter (four clinical sites) prospective trial, involving 326 patients with a history of bladder cancer, evaluated the performance of the ImmunoCyt for the detection of recurrent tumor [9]. Overall sensitivity and specificity were 81 and 75%, respectively. Interestingly, the test appeared to have similar sensitivity irrespective of tumor grade or stage [i.e., low grade: 22/28 (79%); intermediate grade: 9/10 (90%); high grade: 4/6 (67%); carcinoma in situ: 5/5 (100%); Ta: 29/35 (83%); T1: 6/8 (75%); T2: 2/2 (100%)]. In addition, the ImmunoCyt test detected 12 of 17 (71%) small (<1 cm) tumors, whereas cytology could do 3 of them (18%). Previous studies have also suggested the possibility of reducing the frequency of cystoscopies for monitoring patients with low-risk bladder cancer on the basis of ImmunoCyt results [9]. As disadvantages, this test requires significant experience and constant quality control. Nonetheless, the ImmunoCyt test is clearly superior to conventional urine cytology and is likely one of the most promising bladder cancer markers.

UroVysion

Frequent alterations in chromosomes, such as 3, 4, 7, 8, 9, 10, 11, 13, 14, 17, and 18, have been identified in urothelial cancers. Among these, the loss of 9p where the *p16* gene is located (9p21) is most ubiquitously (>50%) found in bladder cancer, although *p16* gene mutations are infrequent. These chromosomal alterations can be easily detected by fluorescence in situ hybridization (FISH). The UroVysion™ (Abbott Molecular Inc, Des Plaines, Illinois) is a multiprobe/multicolor FISH assay kit that detects aneuploidy for chromosomes 3 (red), 7 (green), and 17 (aqua), as well as loss of the 9p21

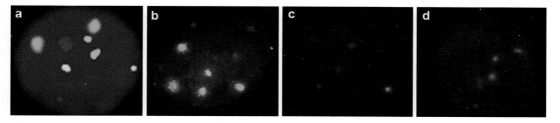

Fig. 7.3 UroVysion (Abbott Molecular Inc.). A multiprobe/multicolor FISH assay kit detecting chromosomes 3 (red), 7 (green), and 17 (aqua), and the 9p21 locus (gold). Normal result observed in an interphase cell (**a**). Abnormal result observed in aneusomic interphase cells (**b–d**)

locus (gold), in exfoliated urothelial cells (Fig. 7.3). There are currently no uniform criteria for determining a positive UroVysion test, but several studies have used the following criteria that the assay is considered positive: (1) ≥4 urinary cells with gains of ≥2 chromosomes; (2) ≥12 urinary cells with gain of a single chromosome; or (3) homologous deletion of 9p21 in >10% of epithelial cells [3]. This kit was approved by the FDA in 2005 for initial diagnosis of bladder cancer in patients with hematuria and subsequent monitoring for tumor recurrence in patients previously diagnosed with bladder cancer. As is the case with the ImmunoCyt test, the UroVysion test requires specific equipment (e.g., fluorescence microscope, computer-assisted image analyzing system) and specially trained personnel.

Various case–control studies, using different thresholds, have shown the sensitivity and specificity of the UroVysion test varying from 39 to 92% and from 85 to 100%, respectively [2, 3, 10–12]. These studies reported a lower sensitivity (32–65%) to detect low-grade and/or low-stage bladder tumors, although 9p21 loss has predominantly been identified in such tumors. A recently published prospective study, involving 250 patients, evaluated the UroVysion test for the detection of recurrent bladder cancer and compared with urine cytologic analysis [13]. This study showed that the sensitivity and specificity of FISH, compared with cytology, are 73 vs. 61% and 87 vs. 80%, respectively. Among 148 cases in which initial cystoscopy and cytology were negative, 56 showed a positive FISH test and 9 patients eventually developed recurrent tumor. Therefore, the authors concluded that the UroVysion test has the capacity to resolve equivocal cytologic findings as well as to detect recurrent tumors before cystoscopically visible lesions can be identified. More recent prospective retrospective studies evaluating the UroVysion test in patients with equivocal and/or malignant urine cytology showed similar sensitivity. Thus, the UroVysion test appears to be a promising bladder cancer marker that may identify both low-grade and high-grade tumors. The uniform criteria used for the evaluation of abnormal cells need to be established.

Potential Markers in Earlier Phases of Clinical Development

Bladder Cancer Antigen-4 (BLCA-4)

BLCA-4 is an NMP and is now known to be a member of the ETS transcription factor family. It expresses in histologically normal bladder tissue, as well as in tumor, in patients with bladder cancer, but not in bladder tissue without bladder cancer. Several clinical trials, using a sandwich ELISA assay which detects BLCA-4 in urine samples, showed high sensitivities (95–96%) and specificities (95–100%) for bladder cancer [2, 3]. It is noted that there were only a few false-positive results in cases with benign urologic conditions. An ongoing large multicenter clinical trial [3] might validate the usefulness of this marker.

Survivin

Survivin is an antiapoptotic protein that functions via blocking caspase activation as well as regulating chromosome alignment and segregation. It has been shown to be highly expressed in a variety of human tumors, including urothelial carcinoma. Recent studies, using quantitative reverse transcription-polymerase chain reaction (RT-PCR), showed that survivin expression in bladder cancer correlates with tumor recurrence and disease-specific mortality [2, 14]. An initial clinical study involving a relatively small number of bladder cancer patients showed a sensitivity of 100% for survivin detected by a dot blot assay (Bio-Dot microfiltration detection system; Bio-Rad, Hercules, California) or RT-PCR in urine. In this study the specificity of survivin was 100% among healthy volunteers and 87% among patients with benign genitourinary disease. A subsequent study analyzing voided urine from 117 bladder cancer patients and 92 controls showed that the survivin dot blot assay had a sensitivity of 64% and a specificity of 93%, which were superior to both conventional cytology and the NMP22 test. A more recent study involving 153 patients with bladder cancer showed a better sensitivity (90%) and specificity (95%) [15]. Splicing variants of survivin for the detection of bladder cancer were also assessed, showing lower sensitivity and/or specificity than those of survivin.

UBC Tests

The UBC™ tests (i.e., UBC-II ELISA, UBC-IRMA; IDL Biotech, Bromma, Sweden) are a monoclonal assay that measures the reactivity against defined epitope structures on cytokeratin (CK) 8 and CK18 in urine samples. European studies evaluating the UBC tests for the detection of primary or recurrent bladder cancer have shown the sensitivity of 35–79% and the specificity of 68–92% [3]. The specificity was particularly low (13–25%) in low-grade/low-stage tumors. Some of these studies also showed that the UBC tests had a lower sensitivity than other markers, including cytology. A recent prospective study involving 166 individuals reported that the UBC-ELISA test has a sensitivity of 40% and a specificity of 75%, both of which are still lower than those of urine cytology (71 and 84%, respectively) [16].

CYFRA 21-1

CYFRA 21-1 is a soluble fragment of CK19 and its levels in urine can be measured by commercially available kits, ELSA CYFRA 21-1 (sandwich immunoradiometric assay; Cisbio International, Cère, France) and ElecSys 2010 system (electrochemiluminescence immunoassay Roche Diagnositics, Indianapolis, Indiana). Previous studies, using different cutoff values of urinary CYFRA 21-1, showed the sensitivity ranging from 75 to 97% and the specificity ranging from 67 to 87% to detect bladder cancer. High levels of CYFRA 21-1 were detected in patients with benign conditions, such as urolithiasis, urinary tract infection, and prostatic hyperplasia. In a recent retrospective study analyzing urine samples from 100 patients with bladder cancer and 50 patients with hematuria but not bladder cancer, the sensitivity of CYFRA 21-1 (74%) was higher than those of telomerase activity (71%), VEGF (69%), and cytology (38%) (also see below) [17]. By contrast, in this study, the specificities of CYFRA 21-1, telomerase, VEGF, and cytology were 78, 84, 88, and 92%, respectively. Other recent studies involving >150 patients with a history of superficial bladder cancer revealed a lower sensitivity of CYFRA 21-1 than previously reported data.

Hyaluronic Acid (HA)-Hyaluronidase (HAase)

HA, a glycosaminoglycan that promotes metastasis, has been shown to be elevated in several human malignancies, including bladder cancer. HAase, an enzyme that degrades HA, has also been detected in urine from patients with bladder cancer. The HA-HAase test is a combination of two ELISA-like assays that measure urinary levels of HA and HAase (the test kit is not commercially available) [1]. This test has been considered positive when either or both assays are positive. In a limited number of studies, the sensitivity of the HA-HAase test for the detection of bladder cancer, regardless of tumor grade, ranged from 83 to 94% (low grade: 75–91%; intermediate grade: 84–100%; high grade: 92–100%) [1–3]. The overall specificity in these studies among individuals with or without a history of bladder cancer and with or without benign urologic disease was 70–84%. In one of the studies [1], a false-positive test in patients with a history of bladder cancer indicated four- to tenfold increased risk of recurrence within 5 months. Furthermore, a recent study measuring HA levels in urine samples from patients with bladder cancer before and after transurethral resection of the tumor suggested that a high level of HA predicts the presence of a residual tumor, with a sensitivity of 93% and a specificity of 83% [18].

Telomerase

Telomerase regenerates telomeres at the end of each DNA replication and sets the molecular clock to immortality. Relative telomerase activity can be assessed by PCR-based telomerase repeat amplification protocol (TRAP) assay, as well as by two alternatives, telomerase RNA template expression and telomerase RT (catalytic subunit) mRNA by RT-PCR. Increased telomerase activity is detected in normal tissue, such as germ cells, and a variety of neoplasms, including almost all cases of bladder cancer. Telomerase activity in urine from patients with bladder cancer, using TRAP assay or RT-PCR, has also been examined [2, 3, 16]. These studies showed wide-ranging sensitivities (9–100%, mostly 70–90%) and specificity (24–99%, mostly >60%) of telomerase activity to detect bladder tumors. Some disadvantages of these methods include false-positivity in benign urologic conditions or benign cells (e.g., lymphocyte) and, for TRAP assay, necessity of at least 50 cells expressing telomerase. Eissa et al. [19] compared the above three methods plus urine cytology to detect bladder cancer. Overall the sensitivity of telomerase RT (by real-time RT-PCR) was the highest compared to that of telomerase RNA (by RT-PCR), relative telomerase activity (by TRAP assay), and cytology (96, 92, 75, and 75%, respectively). Similarly, the specificities of these are 96, 89, 75, and 94%, respectively. The authors concluded that the best combination is telomerase RNA and telomerase RT RNA, but telomerase RNA alone is the most cost-effective method. Some controversies, such as stability of telomerase in exfoliated urothelial cells and discrepancy of activity between voided urine and bladder washing, need to be further investigated.

Quanticyt

Quanticyt is an automated karyometric analysis, using a personal computer-based image analysis system, which measures mean nuclear shape and DNA content in light microscopy images. Currently, this system is not commercially available. The test may be inadequate when there are too few urothelial cells or too many red blood cells/white blood cells. Most of clinical studies evaluating the Quanticyt test for detecting bladder cancer in urine samples have been published by the same group in the Netherlands. The most recent study demonstrated that overall sensitivity and specificity were 42 and 68%, respectively, for the Quanticyt test, compared to those of 41 and 90% for urine cytology and 39 and 90% for the UroVysion test [11]. In a study by another group [20], the Quanticyt test had a sensitivity of 59 and a specificity of 93%, which were equivalent to or better than those of urine cytology (59 and 100%, respectively), BTA test (57 and 68%, respectively), or NMP22 test (48 and 70%, respectively).

Fibroblast Growth Factor Receptor 3 (FGFR3)

Activating somatic point mutations in the *FGFR3* gene are frequently observed in urothelial carcinoma, particularly low-grade tumors. These can be detected in both bladder cancer tissue and voided urine from patients with a tumor by a labor-intensive single-strand conformation polymorphism-sequencing analysis. A PCR-based technique (i.e., SNaPshot mutation assay) in urine for the detection of FGFR3 mutations at nine common sites was reported, showing a sensitivity of 62% and a specificity of 89%. Miyake et al. [21] recently detected FGFR3 mutations in 11 of 13 (85%) urine samples from patients with superficial bladder cancer but in none of the tissues and/or urine samples from patients with invasive bladder cancer or chronic cystitis, using a peptide nucleic acid-mediated real-time PCR clamping method. More recently, FGFR3 mutations were shown to correlate with a concomitant or future recurrence during surveillance of patients presenting with a low-grade tumor [21, 22].

Mucin 7 (MUC7)

Mucins are glycoproteins synthesized by glandular epithelial cells and function, in the bladder, as a selective barrier for urothelium. Among 9 human mucin genes, MUC7 was reported to be up-regulated in invasive bladder carcinoma, compared to low-grade tumor or benign bladder. Two studies published in 2003 evaluated MUC7 for the detection of bladder cancer in exfoliated cells in urine from 50–65 patients, using RT-PCR. Overall sensitivity and specificity of MUC7 were 65–66% and 80–87%, respectively, with a higher sensitivity in high-grade/invasive tumors. A recent study involving 153 patients confirmed these findings by showing a sensitivity of 63% and a specificity of 75% for MUC7, which were additionally compared to those of urine cytology (46 and 100%, respectively) or survivin (90 and 95%, respectively) [14]. However, further confirmation is still necessary to conclude the performance of MUC7 for bladder cancer detection.

VEGF

VEGF is an important regulator of angiogenesis involved in tumor growth, invasion, and metastasis. Increased expression of VEGF in bladder cancer tissue as well as in urine from the patients detected by ELISA assay has been reported. Recent control studies evaluated VEGF as a urine-based bladder cancer marker and compared with urine cytology [2, 16, 23]. Overall sensitivity and specificity of VEGF were 68–77% and 62–93%, respectively, showing higher sensitivity and lower specificity than cytology in all the studies. There was also a tendency that urinary VEGF more reliably identified high-grade or high-stage tumors. However, these studies have used different cutoff points. More cohort studies are necessary to evaluate this marker.

Markers Detected by Immunocytochemistry

Immunochemistry can be applied to formalin-fixed and paraffin-embedded tissue (i.e., cytologic cell blocks), cytologic direct smears, and liquid-based preparations (e.g., ThinPrep and SurePath). Details of immunochemistry, including the utility of major markers in cytology, were previously described in Chapter 45 in Diagnostic Cytology and Its Histopathologic Bases (Koss LG and Melamed MR, Lippincott Williams & Wilkins, 2006). Herein, I highlight several established and novel immunomarkers utilized in detecting urothelial neoplasms and distinguishing those from other benign or malignant conditions.

CKs

CKs are a family of intracytoplasmic intermediate filament proteins present in almost all epithelia. Expression of each CK molecule depends on cell type and differentiation status and, therefore, specific CKs can be used as markers to identify particular types of epithelial tumors. Specifically, immunoprofile of CK7 and CK20 stains is helpful in differentiating the origin of carcinomas. CK7 is found in a wide variety of non-neoplastic epithelia, including urothelium, but not in most gastrointestinal epithelium, hepatocytes, proximal and distal tubules of the kidney, and squamous epithelium. In contrast, CK20 shows relatively restricted expression and is present in gastrointestinal epithelium, Merkel cells of the epidermis, and umbrella cells of urothelium.

Although CK7 expression is observed in the majority of urothelial carcinoma, there are few reports investigating CK7 as an immunomarker in urine samples. CK20 staining on smears from urine specimens was shown to be strong in 12 of 14 (86%) urothelial carcinomas and in 5 of 5 (100%) cases with atypical cytology that were confirmed as carcinoma by following surgery, whereas it was negative in all the 14 benign cases except some umbrella cells with weak stains [24]. Another study staining CK20 in urine of 90 patients (54 carcinomas and 36 controls) demonstrated a sensitivity of 70% and a specificity of 83% [25]. Although the specificity of CK20 expression was lower than that of urine cytology (76%) or ImmunoCyt (83%), simultaneous use of these three markers (93%) was more sensitive than any single marker or a combination of any two (up to 89%). A diagnostic pitfall in CK immunostaining includes occasional AE1/AE3 expression in muscularis propria. Thus, particularly when examining residual tumor cells with CK in patients who underwent a recent surgery, one should pay attention to cytologic appearance of cells. In addition, inflammatory myofibroblastic tumor of the urinary tract in two thirds of which ALK-1 staining is positive occasionally expresses CK.

p53

The tumor suppressor gene $p53$ plays a key role in transcriptional regulation of cell cycle and its mutations represent the most common genetic alterations in human malignancies. A number of studies have revealed $p53$ gene mutations in 40–60% of invasive bladder cancers and their association with a poorer prognosis. Indeed, detection of mutant p53 in the urine of patients with bladder cancer has been being investigated. The altered protein products of the mutant gene that possess extended half-life can be detected in immunohistochemical techniques.

In urine cytology specimens, p53 may be useful as a marker for neoplastic change, particularly in lower-grade tumors where the morphologic changes of neoplasia are subtle. In one such study on urinary specimens processed by filter imprint technique [26], overall p53 positivity in bladder cancer cases was 34%. In 55% of samples, mainly from cases of higher-grade carcinoma with definitive neoplastic cytology, p53 was positive, whereas 23% of cases that were cytologically negative but showed cancer on histological examination of biopsy specimens were p53 positive. The positivity of p53 did not appear to significantly correlate with tumor grade, although 40% of grades 2–3 were positive compared with 21% of grade 1 tumors. A recent study showed an overall p53 positivity in 33 (83%) of 40 bladder cancer cases, including 27 G1, 1 G2, and 5 G3 tumors [27]. In this study, no p53 immunoreactivity was found in control samples.

Ki-67

The Ki-antigen is detected by immunohistochemistry using a monoclonal antibody to MIB-1 that accumulates in the nuclei of proliferating cells from G1 phase to mitosis, but not in resting cells. Several studies have demonstrated the value of Ki-67 as an independent prognostic marker for recurrence and progression of urothelial carcinoma. A study showed that the amounts of Ki-67 RNA in urine from patients with bladder cancer were associated with the protein labeling index of tumor material [28].

p16

p16 is a tumor suppressor gene that inhibits cyclin D-dependent protein kinases and plays a vital role in regulation of G1-S transition. Chromosome 9p21 at which the genes encoding p16 and p15 are localized is frequently involved in heterozygous and homozygous deletions in bladder cancer. As described, these 9p21 deletions, as well as p16/p15 mutations, are more frequently seen in low-grade/superficial tumors than in high-grade/invasive tumors. Immunohistochemical detection of p16 protein has not been widely used in the diagnosis of urothelial carcinoma. Several recent studies showed that there is a significant correlation between loss of p16 expression and poorer outcome in patients with non-muscle invasive disease. In contrast, increased expression of p16 protein in carcinoma in situ, compared to uniform and weak expression in normal or reactive urothelium, was reported. In a study analyzing urine cytologic samples [29], frequent (80%) p16 overexpression was seen in high-grade carcinoma. Rare overexpression of p16 was found in non-neoplastic urothelium.

Epidermal Growth Factor Receptor (EGFR)

Epidermal growth factor and its receptor (EGFR) are key factors in modulating cell proliferation via stimulation of protein-tyrosine kinase activity. Overexpression of EGFR in bladder neoplasms is common and correlates with their malignant potential [2]. EGFR and proliferating cell nuclear antigen (PCNA) expression has been studied in bladder cancer utilizing urine specimens processed as ThinPrep [30]. There were no significant associations between EGFR/PCNA and tumor grade. However, EGFR expression, but not PCNA, was found to be a significant predictor of tumor stage.

E-Cadherin

E-cadherin is a cell-adhesion molecule that has been associated with invasion and metastasis of various malignancies. Although decreased E-cadherin expression is observed in higher stages of bladder cancer, the expression is known to be higher in urothelial carcinoma than in benign urothelium. In a pilot study, 21 (100%) of 21 cytology samples from patients with biopsy-proven carcinoma and 10 (53%) of 19 benign cases showed increased E-cadherin levels over background squamous cell staining [31]. Thus, E-cadherin overexpression can be detected in urine cytology specimens DD23.

The murine IgG monoclonal antibody DD23 recognizes a protein dimer of 185 kDa expressing in human bladder cancer cells. In a study by Sawczuk et al. involving 308 bladder cytology specimens [32], DD23 expression had a sensitivity of 81%, which was enhanced to 85% when combined with cytologic findings, and a specificity of 60% (vs. 85% in cytology only). The same group also evaluated DD23 for the detection of recurrent tumor. Analysis of 64 cases of biopsy-proven recurrent urothelial carcinoma yielded sensitivities of 70 and 44% and specificities of 60 and 92% for DD23 and cytology, respectively. When these two were combined, the sensitivity was increased to 78%. Interestingly, DD23 enhanced the sensitivity from 20% (cytology alone) to 55% for low-grade tumors and from 64% (cytology alone) to 76% for high-grade tumors. Furthermore, DD23 did not apparently lose sensitivity in patients who underwent intravesical therapy after initial surgery. Thus, DD23 antigen expression can be used as an adjunct to cytopathologic evaluation to enhance the sensitivity of urinary cytology detection of urothelial carcinoma.

Comparison Between Urine Cytology and FDA-Approved Markers

Many studies have compared various potential bladder cancer markers with each other and with conventional urine cytology. As described, in most of markers, the sensitivity varies with tumor grade and stage. Moreover, the specificity was influenced by the population of control group (e.g., false-positive results in patients with benign genitourinary conditions). Table 7.1 summarizes some of comparative studies that assess the sensitivity and specificity of FDA-approved markers and cytology. These markers have a higher overall sensitivity but a lower overall specificity than cytology to detect bladder cancer. Van Rhijn et al. [33] also reviewed 64 articles of comparative analysis of bladder cancer markers and showed similar results for tumor surveillance. These studies suggest that non-invasive tests

Table 7.1 The sensitivity and specificity for urine cytology and FDA-approved bladder cancer markers from comparative studies

| Study (year) [Ref.] | Sensitivity (%)/specificity (%) | | | | | |
	Cytology	BTA	NMP22	ImmunoCyt	UroVysion	FDP
Landman et al. (1998)	40/94	40/73	81/77			
Ramakumar et al. (1998)	44/95	74/73	53/60			
Wiener et al. (1998) [20]	59/100	57/68	48/69			
Del Nero et al. (1999)	54/100	54/70	91/77			
Sharma et al. (1999)	56/93	68/82	82/82			
Sözen et al. (1999)	35/90	69/68	73/85			
Giannopoulos et al. (2001)	39/94	72/57	63/74			
Messing et al. (2005) [9]	23/93			81/75		
Têtu et al. (2005) [7]	29/98			74/62		
Mian et al. (2006) [8]	39/99			85/73		
Placer et al. (2002) [10]	64/86				80/85	
Moonen et al. (2007) [12]	41/90				39/90	
Yoder et al. (2007) [13]	61/80				73/87	
Sullivan et al. (2009)	21/97			76/63	13/90	
van Rhijn et al.[a] (2005) [33]	48/94	58[b],71[c]/73[b],66[c]	71/73	67/75	79/70	54/61

[a] A review article showing the median sensitivity/specificity
[b] BTA-stat test
[c] BTA-TRAK test

currently used in a surveillance setting, in combination with urine cytology, may be able to reduce the frequency of invasive cystoscopic examination.

In addition to potential clinical benefits, the cost for each test needs to be considered to assess its economic impact. The POC tests, such as BTA and NMP22, are inexpensive ($20–40/test). In contrast, the tests requiring specialized labs, including ImmunoCyt and UroVysion, cost at least $200 (up to $900), which could be even more expensive than the standard care with urine cytology and cystoscopy (approximately $400). Nonetheless, if a positive result of a marker leads to avoidance of more expensive and invasive tests, such as a biopsy, the marker could still be cost-effective.

Conclusion

Urine cytology, in conjunction with cystoscopic examination, remains the standard procedure in the evaluation of bladder lesions to rule out neoplasms. Conventional cytologic analysis has a very high specificity in detecting urothelial carcinoma, but is not sensitive, especially in low-grade tumors. Due to the limitation of urine cytology as well as the costly and invasive nature of cystoscopy, much research has been directed to develop urinary markers for non-invasively detecting bladder cancer. Indeed, many of the current markers have higher sensitivities than, with comparable specificities to, cytology. Thus, these tests could be a useful adjunct for cytology and cystoscopy. In addition, some of them have been shown to have prognostic value in patients with urothelial carcinoma. Nonetheless, at least in the near future, complete elimination of cystoscopy and/or cytology for the detection and surveillance of carcinomas is unlikely feasible. Accordingly, additional non-invasive tests may still need to be identified. Cost-effectiveness of the markers is also to be investigated further.

References

1. Lokeshwar VB, Schroeder GL, Selzer MG, et al. Bladder tumor markers for monitoring recurrence and screening comparison of hyaluronic acid-hyaluronidase and BTA-Stat tests. Cancer. 2002;95:61–72.
2. Vrooman OPJ, Witjes JA. Molecular markers for detection, surveillance and prognostication of bladder cancer. Int J Urol. 2009;16:234–43.
3. Lokeshwar VB, Habuchi T, Grossman HB, et al. Bladder tumor markers beyond cytology: international consensus panel on bladder tumor markers. Urology. 2005;66(Suppl 6A):35–63.
4. Grossman HB, Messing E, Soloway M, et al. Detection of bladder cancer using a point-of-care proteomic assay. JAMA. 2005;293:810–6.
5. Grossman HB, Soloway M, Messing E, et al. Surveillance for recurrent bladder cancer using a point-of-care proteomic assay. JAMA. 2006;295:299–305.
6. Topsakal M, Karadeniz T, Anaç M, Dönmezer S, Besisik A. Assessment of fibrin-fibrinogen degradation products (Accu-Dx) test in bladder cancer patients. Eur Urol. 2001;39:287–91.
7. Têtu B, Tiguert R, Harel F, Fradet Y. ImmunoCyt/uCyt+™ improves the sensitivity of urine cytology in patients followed for urothelial carcinoma. Mod Pathol. 2005;18:83–9.
8. Mian C, Maier K, Comploj E, et al. uCyt+/ImmunoCyt™ in the detection of recurrent urothelial carcinoma: An update on 1991 analyses. Cancer. 2006;108:60–5.
9. Messing EM, Teot L, Korman H, et al. Performance of urine test in patients monitored for recurrence of bladder cancer: a multicenter study in the United States. J Urol. 2005;174:1238–41.
10. Placer J, Espinet B, Salido M, Solé F, Gelabert-Mas A. Clinical utility of a multiprobe FISH assay in voided urine specimens for the detection of bladder cancer and its recurrences, compared with urine cytology. Eur Urol. 2002;42:547–52.
11. Laudadio J, Keane TE, Reeves HM, Savage SJ, Hoda RS, Lage JM, Wolff DJ. Fluorescence in situ hybridization for detecting transitional cell carcinoma: implications for clinical practice. BJU Int. 2005;96:1280–5.
12. Moonen PM, Merkx GF, Peelen P, Karthaus HF, Smeets DF, Witjes JA. UroVysion compared with cytology and quantitative cytology in the surveillance of non-muscle-invasive bladder cancer. Eur Urol. 2007;51:1275–80.

13. Yoder BJ, Skacel M, Hedgepeth R, et al. Reflex UroVysion testing of bladder cancer surveillance patients with equivocal or negative urine cytology: a prospective study with focus on the natural history of anticipatory positive findings. Am J Clin Pathol. 2007;127:295–301.

14. Shariat SF, Ashfaq R, Karakiewicz PI, Saeedi O, Sagalowsky AI, Lotan Y. Survivin expression is associated with bladder cancer presence, stage, progression, and mortality. Cancer. 2007;109:1106–13.

15. Pu X-Y, Wang Z-P, Chen Y-R, Wang X-H, Wu Y-L, Wang H-P. The value of combined use of survivin, cytokeratin 20 and mucin 7 mRNA for bladder cancer detection in voided urine. J Cancer Res Clin Oncol. 2008;134:659–65.

16. May M, Hakenberg OW, Gunia S, et al. Comparative diagnostic value of urine cytology, UBC-ELISA, and fluorescence in situ hybridization for detection of transitional cell carcinoma of urinary bladder in routine clinical practice. Urology. 2007;70:449–53.

17. Bian W, Xu Z. Combined assay of CYFRA21-1, telomerase and vascular endothelial growth factor in the detection of bladder transitional cell carcinoma. Int J Urol. 2007;14:108–11.

18. Passerotti CC, Bonfim A, Martins JR, et al. Urinary hyaluronan as a marker for the presence of residual transitional cell carcinoma of the urinary bladder. Eur Urol. 2006;49:71–5.

19. Eissa S, Swellam M, Ali-Labib R, Mansour A, El-Malt O, Tash FM. Detection of telomerase in urine by 3 methods: evaluation of diagnostic accuracy for bladder cancer. J Urol. 2007;178:1668–72.

20. Wiener HG, Mian C, Haitel A, Pycha A, Schatzl G, Marberger M. Can urine bound diagnostic tests replace cystoscopy in the management of bladder cancer? J Urol. 1998;159:1876–80.

21. Miyake M, Sugano K, Kawashima K, et al. Sensitive detection of FGFR3 mutations in bladder cancer and urine sediments by peptide nucleic acid-mediated real-time PCR clamping. Biochem Biophys Res Commun. 2007;362:865–71.

22. Zuiverloon TC, van der Aa MN, van der Kwast TH, et al. Fibroblast growth factor receptor 3 mutation analysis on voided urine for surveillance of patients with low-grade non-muscle-invasive bladder cancer. Clin Cancer Res. 2010;16:3011–8.

23. Eissa S, Salem AM, Zohny SF, Hegazy MGA. The diagnostic efficacy of urinary TGF-β1 and VEGF in bladder cancer: comparison with voided urine cytology. Cancer Biomark. 2007;3:275–85.

24. Bhatia A, Dey P, Kumar Y, et al. Expression of cytokeratin 20 in urine cytology smears: a potential marker for the detection of urothelial carcinoma. Cytopathology. 2007;18:84–6.

25. Soyuer I, Sofikerim M, Tokat F, Soyuer S, Ozturk F. Which urine marker test provides more diagnostic value in conjunction with standard cytology-ImmunoCyt/uCyt+ or cytokeratin 20 expression. Diagn Pathol. 2009;4:20.

26. Righi E, Rossi G, Ferrari G, et al. Does p53 immunostaining improve diagnostic accuracy in urine cytology? Diagn Cytopathol. 1997;17:436–9.

27. Oğuztüzün S, Sezgin Y, Yazici S, Firat P, Özhavzali M, Özen H. Expression of glutathione-S-transferases isoenzymes and P53 in exfoliated human bladder cancer cells. Urol Oncol. 2011;29:538–44.

28. Menke TB, Boettcher K, Krüger S, et al. Ki-67 protein concentrations in urothelial bladder carcinomas are related to Ki-67-specific RNA concentrations in urine. Clin Chem. 2004;50:1461–3.

29. Nakazawa K, Murata S-i, Yuminamochi T. p16^{INK4a} expression analysis as an ancillary tool for cytologic diagnosis of urothelial carcinoma. Am J Clin Pathol. 2009;132:776–84.

30. Politi EN, Lazaris AC, Lambropoulou S, Alexopoulou D, Kyriakidou V, Koutselini H. Epidermal growth factor receptor and proliferating cell nuclear antigen expression in urine ThinPrep specimens. Cytopathology. 2005;16:303–8.

31. Ross JS, Cheung C, Sheehan C, del Rosario AD, Bui HX, Fisher HA. E-cadherin cell-adhesion molecule expression as a diagnostic adjunct in urothelial cytology. Diagn Cytopathol. 1996;14:310–5.

32. Sawczuk IS, Pickens CL, Vasa UR, et al. DD23 biomarker: a prospective clinical assessment in routine urinary cytology specimens from patients being monitored for TCC. Urol Oncol. 2002;7:185–90.

33. van Rhijn BWG, van der Poel HG, van der Kwast TH. Urine markers for bladder cancer surveillance: a systematic review. Eur Urol. 2005;47:736–48.

Index

L.G. Koss and R.S. Hoda, *Koss's Cytology of the Urinary Tract with Histopathologic Correlations*,
DOI 10.1007/978-1-4614-2056-9, © Leopold G. Koss 2012

Printed in the United States of America